Questions and Answers
for the
MFSRH

Questions and Answers for the MFSRH

Paula Briggs MB ChB, FFSRH

Southport and Ormskirk Hospital NHS Trust

Tina Dwivedi MBBS, MFSRH

East Lancashire Hospitals NHS Trust

Melisa Thomas MB ChB, MRCOG, DFSRH

North West Deanery

Scion

© **Scion Publishing Limited, 2018**

ISBN 9781911510185

First published 2018

A CIP catalogue record for this book is available from the British Library.

Scion Publishing Limited

The Old Hayloft, Vantage Business Park, Bloxham Road, Banbury OX16 9UX, UK

www.scionpublishing.com

Important Note from the Publisher

The information contained within this book was obtained by Scion Publishing Ltd from sources believed by us to be reliable. However, while every effort has been made to ensure its accuracy, no responsibility for loss or injury whatsoever occasioned to any person acting or refraining from action as a result of information contained herein can be accepted by the authors or publishers.

Readers are reminded that medicine is a constantly evolving science and while the authors and publishers have ensured that all dosages, applications and practices are based on current indications, there may be specific practices which differ between communities. You should always follow the guidelines laid down by the manufacturers of specific products and the relevant authorities in the country in which you are practising.

Although every effort has been made to ensure that all owners of copyright material have been acknowledged in this publication, we would be pleased to acknowledge in subsequent reprints or editions any omissions brought to our attention.

Registered names, trademarks, etc. used in this book, even when not marked as such, are not to be considered unprotected by law.

Typeset by Phoenix Photosetting, Chatham, Kent, UK

Printed in the UK by Ashford Colour Press

Last digit is the print number: 10 9 8 7 6 5 4 3 2 1

Contents

Preface

The Membership examination for the Faculty of Sexual and Reproductive Health, part of the RCOG, is a three part process. Several years ago, MFSRH replaced MFFP. Candidates must sit and pass Part One and undertake and pass an Evidence Based Commentary, before they are eligible for Part Two of the examination.

A revision course for Part Two of the exam was delivered in Liverpool in 2016, with the majority of candidates for the exam that year attending. The feedback was excellent, but a resounding issue was lack of an available text to support preparation for the exam.

This was the incentive to develop this revision guide.

The book includes background information regarding both Part One and Part Two of the exam and sample questions for all parts of the membership examination. Candidates must continue to access current information from the FSRH website and observe the recommended reading lists. It is important to state that this handbook has been developed independently from the FSRH. It is, however, hoped that this text will fill some of the gaps.

Good luck with your exams!

Paula Briggs, Melisa Thomas and Tina Dwivedi

January 2018

Abbreviations

ALOs	actinomyces-like organisms
ART	antiretroviral therapy
BMI	body mass index
BV	bacterial vaginosis
CBT	cognitive behavioural therapy
CHC	combined hormonal contraceptive
CIN	cervical intraepithelial neoplasia
COC	combined oral contraceptive
COPD	chronic obstructive pulmonary disease
CRL	crown rump length
CRP	C-reactive protein
Cu-IUD	copper intrauterine device
EC	emergency contraception
EVAC	evacuation
FGM	female genital mutilation
FSH	follicle stimulating hormone
GnRH	gonadotrophin releasing hormone
GTD	gestational trophoblastic disease
hCG	human chorionic gonadotrophin
HIV	human immunodeficiency virus
HPV	human papillomavirus
HRT	hormone replacement therapy
IBS	irritable bowel syndrome
ICE	Ideas, Concerns, Expectations
ICU	intensive care unit
IUC	intrauterine contraception
IUD	intrauterine device
IUS	intrauterine system
IVF	*in vitro* fertilisation
LAPCM	long acting permanent contraceptive methods
LARC	long acting reversible methods of contraception
LH	luteinising hormone
LMP	last menstrual period
LNG-EC	levonorgestrel emergency contraception
LNG-IUS	levonorgestrel-containing intrauterine system
NSAID	non-steroidal anti-inflammatory drug
OHSS	ovarian hyperstimulation syndrome
PALS	Patient Advice and Liaison Service

PCOS	polycystic ovarian syndrome
PEP	post-exposure prophylaxis
PEPSE	PEP following sexual exposure
PMS	premenstrual syndrome
POCT	point of care test
POI	premature ovarian insufficiency
POP	progestogen-only pill
PPH	postpartum haemorrhage
PrEP	pre-exposure prophylaxis
SLE	systemic lupus erythematosus
SPC	specific product characteristic
SSRI	selective serotonin reuptake inhibitor
STI	sexually transmitted infection
UI	urge incontinence
UKMEC	UK Medical Eligibility Criteria
UPA-EC	ulipristal acetate emergency contraception
UPSI	unprotected sexual intercourse
UTI	urinary tract infection
VIN	vulval intraepithelial neoplasia
VTE	venous thromboembolism

PART
ONE

Introduction to MFSRH Part One

Introduction to MFSRH Part One

Part One of the MFSRH exam is aimed to assess trainees at ST3 level and involves answering 60 questions in 90 minutes. The questions take the format of 'single best answer' (SBA) in which you need to pick the single best answer out of 5 possible answers. Part One MFSRH is set out to test your applied clinical knowledge and so the majority of the questions will be based on a clinical vignette.

To guide your revision, it is essential that you familiarise yourself with the 'Syllabus for MFSRH Part One' which is in the 'MFSRH Part One Handbook' found on the FSRH website (www.fsrh.org).

The curriculum modules covered by MFSRH Part One are:

- **Module 2:** Contraception
- **Module 3:** Unplanned pregnancy and abortion care
- **Module 4:** Gynaecology (medical and surgical)
- **Module 5:** Speciality gynaecology (subfertility, oncology, urogynaecology)
- **Module 6:** Pregnancy (antenatal, intrapartum, postnatal)
- **Module 7:** Menopause and premenstrual syndrome
- **Module 8:** Genitourinary medicine
- **Module 13:** Information technology, audit and research

The 'MFSRH Part One Handbook' also includes a reading list and this is an invaluable list of resources on which questions for the exam are based.

The modified Angoff standard setting method is used to determine the pass mark for each exam. Therefore, the pass mark will vary between exams depending on the difficulty of the questions set.

Hints and tips to help you succeed in MFSRH Part One

1. **Start early and make a revision timetable**
   You don't want to have to re-sit this exam so preparation is essential. Most of you are working full time, and have family and social commitments to fit alongside revising and so it is important that you organise your time. Make a revision timetable, as this will keep you focused and allow you to build in time for relaxing which is vital to make sure you don't burn out.

2. **Talk to your colleagues**
   Your colleagues have been in your position and none of them will have forgotten what it feels like. Use your colleagues, especially those who have sat the exam recently. They will be able to advise you what resources they found useful and how they managed their time.

3. **Get a study buddy**
   When you start looking through the reading list and curriculum you will realise that there is a lot to cover. Working with someone else can save you time and keep you sane. Try summarising a guideline each and discussing it or, even better, write your own questions to highlight the most important points.

4. **Know your guidelines**
   Exam questions are not set out to trick you. The exam is set to make sure you can adapt your knowledge to a clinical situation and to ensure that you are managing patients safely. The majority of the questions are taken from clinical situations and guidelines that you use every day.

5. **Timed practice**
   In the exam, you will need to get through 60 questions in 90 minutes; this gives you 90 seconds per question. When you are doing practice questions try to simulate the exam setting: sit in a quiet room, turn off your phone and time yourself. Using this method of revision will give you a better awareness of time and make you feel more confident on the day of the exam.

6. **Read the question**
   There are two main reasons for this: first, it is easy to get side-tracked by the information in the vignette and miss the point of the question. Secondly, the clues to the answer are in the vignette and you should use this information when answering the question.

7. **Cover the answers**

When you are answering SBAs it is easy to get distracted by the list of answers. One way to avoid this is to read the question but cover the answer options. Write your answer down and uncover the answer options. Use this technique when you are doing your practice papers and you will find that you save time and get less distracted.

8. **Answer all the questions**

The exam is not negatively marked so make sure you don't leave any questions out. You are better giving yourself a 20% chance rather than a 0% chance of getting the answer right.

9. **Be prepared on the day**

Preparation is key. Find out what time the exam is and where it will be. Research transport options or book a hotel the night before. Make sure you have everything you need, and that includes food, a drink and a jumper (exam halls get cold!).

10. **Be positive**

This is most important! When the exam day finally arrives, remember how much you have done to get to this stage and go into the exam prepared with a positive mental attitude.

Practice paper 1: SBA questions

1. You see a 21-year-old woman who is requesting emergency contraception. She reports having unprotected sexual intercourse 24 hours ago. Her BMI is 24, she has epilepsy and is taking phenytoin. You offer her the copper intrauterine device but she refuses it.

    What would be the next most appropriate treatment option?

    a. Ulipristal acetate 30mg

    b. Levonorgestrel 1.5mg

    c. Levonorgestrel 3mg

    d. Insist that she has the Cu-IUD

    e. Ulipristal acetate 60mg

2. You are consenting a patient prior to insertion of an intrauterine contraceptive device.

    What is the risk of uterine perforation during insertion of an IUC?

    a. 2 in 10

    b. 2 in 20

    c. 2 in 50

    d. 2 in 100

    e. 2 in 1000

3. A 32-year-old woman with a BMI of 22 is complaining of vaginal spotting most days. She had a levonorgestrel-containing intrauterine system (LNG-IUS) inserted 10 months ago and she is happy using it for contraception but would like the bleeding to stop. An ultrasound scan has confirmed optimal placement of the device.

    What is the best treatment to manage this patient's symptoms?

    a. Use the progestogen -only pill for 3 months

    b. Use of a combined oral contraceptive for 3 months

    c. Advise her that she should have her LNG-IUS removed and use another form of contraception

    d. Start her on norethisterone 5mg three times a day for 10 days

    e. Change her LNG-IUS to a Cu-IUD

4. Insertion and removal of progestogen-only contraceptive implants is associated with nerve and vascular injury.

   What is the best location to site a progestogen-only implant?

   a. In the groove between the biceps and triceps muscles

   b. 8–10cm above the lateral epicondyle of the humerus

   c. One-third of the way up the arm from the elbow

   d. 8–10cm above the medial epicondyle of the humerus deep to the biceps muscle

   e. Inner side of the upper arm over the biceps muscle

5. You review a 45-year-old patient 3 months after insertion of a 52mg LNG-IUS (Mirena) for contraception and heavy menstrual bleeding. Her bleeding is much lighter. Examination confirms correct placement of the device. The patient would like to know when the device needs to be removed.

   What is the most appropriate advice regarding removal of her LNG-IUS?

   a. Remove device in 3 years

   b. LNG-IUS can be used as contraception up to the age of 55

   c. Remove device in 5 years

   d. Remove device in 10 years

   e. She can use it as endometrial protection up to the age of 55

6. A 51-year-old lady is taking the progestogen-only pill (desogestrel POP). She has been amenorrhoeic on it for the last 3 years. The patient reports experiencing menopausal symptoms over the last year. She wants to know if she can stop her contraceptive pill.

   What is the best advice to give her from the options below?

   a. The POP can be stopped at 50 years of age

   b. Offer to check her FSH levels, if FSH >30IU/L she can stop the POP

   c. Offer to check her FSH levels, if FSH <30IU/L she can stop the POP

   d. Offer to check her FSH levels, if FSH >30IU/L continue POP and re-check FSH in 1 year

   e. Offer to check her FSH levels, if FSH >30IU/L she can stop the POP in 1 year

7. A 35-year-old woman is diagnosed with a miscarriage at 8 weeks. She has minimal bleeding and pain.

    What is the most appropriate management for this patient?

    a. Surgical management of miscarriage

    b. Manual vacuum aspiration

    c. Expectant management of miscarriage

    d. Medical management of miscarriage with 800mcg misoprostol

    e. Medical management of miscarriage with mifepristone and misoprostol

8. A 24-year-old woman attends with an acute onset left-sided pelvic pain. She is haemodynamically stable. Her hCG is 6000IU/L.

    Transvaginal ultrasound: *no intrauterine pregnancy seen. Left adnexal mass 30×35×25mm, moderate free fluid in the rectouterine pouch. Left ovary not visualised, right ovary normal.*

    What is the most appropriate management for this patient?

    a. Admit and repeat the hCG in 48 hours

    b. Discharge with a follow-up hCG in 48 hours

    c. Discuss medical and surgical management of ectopic

    d. Discuss and consent patient for open salpingectomy

    e. Discuss and consent for laparoscopic salpingectomy

9. You are counselling a 30-year-old woman following her first miscarriage. She is upset and anxious.

    What is her age-related risk of miscarriage?

    a. 11%

    b. 12%

    c. 13%

    d. 15%

    e. 20%

10. You review a patient following an early pregnancy USS. The scan reports a 'snowstorm' pattern inside the uterus and bilateral adnexal cysts. The patient has had some vaginal bleeding and is complaining of abdominal bloating and distension. Her LMP is 8 weeks ago and her hCG is 150 000IU/L.

Which of the following is the most likely explanation for the adnexal cysts?

a. Dermoid cysts

b. Endometriomata

c. Corpus luteum cysts

d. Theca lutein cysts

e. Simple cysts

11. An 18-year-old woman underwent an EVAC and the histology confirmed a complete molar pregnancy. During follow-up her hCG fell quickly, with a negative result 3 weeks following the procedure.

What is the recommended follow-up for this patient?

a. 56 days from EVAC

b. 56 days from negative hCG

c. 6 months from EVAC

d. 6 months from negative hCG

e. 12 months in total

12. Aspirin 75mg from 12 weeks of gestation can reduce the risk of pre-eclampsia during pregnancy.

Which one of the following is not an indication for aspirin?

a. Chronic kidney disease

b. Antiphospholipid antibody-positive

c. Diabetes

d. Chronic hypertension

e. Multiple pregnancy

13. A 32-year-old woman is seen at 6 weeks postnatal for a debrief. She developed pre-eclampsia in her last pregnancy. She was induced and delivered at 33+6. She wants to know what her risk of developing pre-eclampsia is in a future pregnancy.

What is the risk of recurrence of pre-eclampsia?

a. 7%

b. 13%

c. 16%

d. 25%

e. 50%

14. A 23-year-old woman attends the assessment unit at 34+5 weeks. She complains of painful genital lesions. On examination, you suspect this is genital herpes. You perform a swab and blood test for antibodies and commence oral aciclovir for 5 days.

    Which one of the following is the most appropriate advice to give her about her delivery?

    a. Delivery by caesarean section

    b. Continue aciclovir in a prophylactic dose and deliver by caesarean section

    c. Aim for vaginal delivery

    d. Prophylactic aciclovir from 36 weeks and a vaginal delivery

    e. Continue prophylactic oral aciclovir and convert to IV during vaginal delivery

15. In the foetal circulation which vessel bypasses the liver to transport oxygenated blood from the placenta to the inferior vena cava?

    a. Foramen ovale

    b. Ductus arteriosus

    c. Ductus venosus

    d. Ligamentum teres

    e. Umbilical vein

16. A 33-year-old woman who is 30 weeks into her first pregnancy attends complaining of vaginal bleeding. On examination, you confirm a minor ante-partum haemorrhage. She has had an uncomplicated pregnancy; her blood group is rhesus B negative and she had her routine anti-D at 28 weeks. She is admitted for observation.

    What is the most appropriate next step?

    a. No need for anti-D as she had her prophylactic dose at 28 weeks

    b. 250IU anti-D

    c. 500IU anti-D

    d. Test for foetal maternal haemorrhage and give 500IU anti-D

    e. Test for foetal maternal haemorrhage and give 1500IU anti-D

17. A 26-year-old woman attends labour ward at 39+5, she reports that her waters broke 1 hour ago and she is contracting 4 times in 10 minutes. This is her first pregnancy. She is known to be a carrier of group B streptococcus. On examination, she is 5cm dilated, her observations and the foetal heart rate are normal.

What is the most appropriate next step?

a. IV co-amoxiclav

b. Oral erythromycin

c. IV benzylpenicillin

d. Take a full blood count and CRP

e. IV clindamycin

18. You are consenting a woman for a caesarean section.

What is the risk of foetal laceration at caesarean section?

a. <1%

b. 1–2%

c. 2–3%

d. 5%

e. 10%

19. You take a phone call from a patient's husband. The woman is 3 days postnatal, he describes her as acting strangely; she appears confused and is shouting out at things that aren't there. She told him that her 3-day-old daughter is communicating with the police and they want to arrest her.

What is the most appropriate next step?

a. Advise him to take her to the GP for immediate assessment

b. Advise them to attend for an urgent appointment with the perinatal mental health team with a view to adult psychiatric ward admission

c. Advise them to book an appointment with the perinatal mental health team

d. Advise them to contact their midwife for assessment

e. Advise them to attend for an urgent appointment with the perinatal mental health team with a view to a mother and baby unit admission

20. A 53-year-old patient presents complaining of vaginal dryness and irritation. You examine her and diagnose atrophic vaginitis. She is on sequential hormone replacement therapy which she started 2 years ago. She has tried over-the-counter lubricants with no effect.

What is the best management for this patient's symptoms?

a. Recommend persevering with lubricants

b. Topical vaginal oestrogen

c. Teach her how to use vaginal dilators

d. Topical local anaesthetic gel

e. 0.05% clobetasone butyrate

21. A 53-year-old woman with a BMI of 24 reports having irregular periods. She has only had one period in the last 12 months which was quite heavy. She is complaining of hot flushes which are worse at night and has recently noticed some pain and dryness during sexual intercourse.

Which one of the following is the most likely diagnosis?

a. Postmenopause

b. Perimenopause

c. Primary ovarian insufficiency

d. Heavy menstrual bleeding

e. Premature menopause

22. What is the average age of the menopause in the UK?

a. 49

b. 50

c. 51

d. 52

e. 53

23. A 35-year-old heavy smoker with a BMI of 36 attends complaining of low mood and irritability the week before her period. This is affecting her relationship with her partner. You suspect she has premenstrual syndrome. You give her lifestyle advice and ask her to complete a symptom diary. Her symptom diary confirms a cyclical pattern to her symptoms.

What is the most appropriate next step in her management?

a. Drospirenone-containing combined oral contraceptive

b. Oestradiol patches 100mcg and micronised progesterone 100mg days 17–28

c. GnRH analogue for 6 months

d. Citalopram 10mg

e. Amitriptyline 25mg

24. A 32-year-old patient with a BMI of 28 diagnosed with premenstrual syndrome has tried lifestyle modification and cognitive behavioural therapy. She is complaining that her symptoms have not improved and she would like to try something else. You want to start her on a combined oral contraceptive.

What is the most appropriate treatment from the options below?

   a. Ethinylestradiol 30mcg / drospirenone 3mg

   b. Ethinylestradiol 30mcg / norethisterone 1.5mg

   c. Ethinylestradiol 30mcg / levonorgestrel 150mcg

   d. Ethinylestradiol 35mcg / norgestimate 75mcg

   e. Ethinylestradiol 30mcg / desogestrel 150mcg

25. What is the first line investigation for premenstrual syndrome?

   a. LH and FSH levels

   b. Oestradiol levels

   c. Trial of GnRH analogue for 3 months

   d. Prospective symptoms diary over two cycles

   e. Prospective symptoms diary over 3 months

26. A 32-year-old woman attends complaining of amenorrhoea for 6 months. She is fit and well with a BMI of 20. Recent blood tests show a raised FSH, normal LH and low oestradiol with normal prolactin.

What is the most likely diagnosis?

   a. Polycystic ovarian syndrome

   b. Pregnancy

   c. Hypogonadotrophic hypogonadism

   d. Hyperprolactinaemia

   e. Premature ovarian insufficiency

27. A 23-year-old with a BMI of 32 attends for fertility investigations. Her partner's semen analysis is normal. A pelvic USS was normal but she reports having irregular periods. Her bloods on Day 2 are:

   LH = 9U/L

   FSH = 3U/L

   Prolactin = 650U/L

   Oestradiol = 86pg/ml

   Testosterone = 2.3nmol/L

What is the most likely diagnosis?

a. Ovarian hyperthecosis

b. Congenital adrenal hyperplasia

c. Polycystic ovarian syndrome

d. Cushing syndrome

e. Turner syndrome

28. A 30-year-old woman is having fertility investigations. Her bloods show that she is ovulating and her partner's semen analysis is normal. An USS pelvis shows normal anteverted uterus, normal ovaries bilateral hydrosalpinx, no free fluid seen. Bilateral tubal occlusion is confirmed during laparoscopy and dye.

What is the next step in this couple's management?

a. Offer IVF

b. Laparoscopic tubal drainage

c. Intrauterine insemination

d. Laparoscopic bilateral salpingectomy followed by IVF

e. Vaginal swabs, oral antibiotics followed by IVF

29. A 34-year-old with no co-morbidities is undergoing fertility investigations. Her bloods and her partner's semen analysis were normal.

What is the most appropriate investigation to assess tubal patency?

a. Laparoscopy and dye

b. Hysterosalpingography

c. USS pelvis

d. Hysteroscopy

e. CT pelvis

30. A 27-year-old man undergoes a semen analysis and is found to have oligozoospermia. His bloods reveal a normal testosterone, low FSH and LH. He lives a healthy lifestyle and enjoys keeping fit.

What is the most likely cause of his oligozoospermia?

a. Kallmann syndrome

b. Exogenous hormones

c. Hyperprolactinaemia

    d. Pituitary insufficiency

    e. Young disease

31. A patient comes to discuss her urinary incontinence. She explains that she leaks urine mainly when she stands up or coughs. She gets occasional dysuria, no haematuria and when she has finished urinating she feels that she needs to go again straight away. Her urinalysis is normal.

What would be your initial investigation?

    a. USS pelvis

    b. Uroflometry

    c. Multi-channel urodynamics

    d. Bladder scan for post-residual volume

    e. U+Es

32. A 56-year-old woman referred by her GP presents complaining of passing urine frequently and an episode of incontinence before reaching the toilet. She is otherwise well.

What is the most appropriate first line investigation?

    a. U+Es

    b. USS pelvis

    c. Pad test

    d. Bladder diary

    e. Urodynamic testing

33. A 51-year-old woman presents with symptoms of stress incontinence.

What first line management would you offer her?

    a. Bladder training for 6 weeks

    b. Supervised pelvic floor muscle training for 3 months

    c. Duloxetine

    d. Oxybutynin

    e. Tolterodine

34. Human papillomavirus has been found to be the leading cause of cervical cancer.

What type of virus is HPV?

    a. Single-stranded RNA

b. Double-stranded RNA

c. Single-stranded DNA

d. Double-stranded DNA

e. Cytomegalovirus

35. Postmenopausal bleeding is associated with endometrial cancer.

What is the most common cause of postmenopausal bleeding?

a. Endometrial polyp

b. Endometrial hyperplasia

c. Endometrial carcinoma

d. Exogenous oestrogens

e. Atrophic endometritis and vaginitis

36. A 57-year-old woman presents with postmenopausal bleeding. She has a BMI of 41. A transvaginal ultrasound scan shows: *retroverted uterus, thickened endometrium with a hyperechoic lesion seen with cystic spaces and an echogenic outline. Normal ovaries, no free fluid in the pelvis.*

What is the most likely cause for her bleeding?

a. Endometrial hyperplasia

b. Endometrial polyp

c. Endometrial cancer

d. Cervical cyst

e. Fibroid

37. What is the risk of progression from endometrial hyperplasia without atypia to endometrial cancer if left untreated?

a. 1%

b. 2%

c. 3%

d. 5%

e. 10%

38. You design a study to compare the BMI of women before and after enrolling on a healthy eating and exercise programme.

What is the most appropriate type of statistical test?

a. Chi-squared

b. Pearson's regression

c. Mann–Whitney U

d. Two sample (unpaired) *t*-test

e. One sample (paired) *t*-test

39. You design a study to compare the mean length of time it takes for the hCG to drop to negative following medical and surgical management of miscarriage.

What is the most appropriate type of statistical test?

a. Chi-squared

b. Pearson's regression

c. Mann–Whitney U

d. Two sample (unpaired) *t*-test

e. One sample (paired) *t*-test

40. Research is an essential part of developing healthcare.

Which of the following is not one of the general ethical principles for medical research?

a. Autonomy

b. Beneficence

c. Non-maleficence

d. Justice

e. Consent

41. We often use the positive predictive value to assess the effectiveness of a screening test.

What is the definition of positive predictive value?

a. The number of patients with a condition having a positive test

b. The number of patients without the condition that have a negative test

c. The number of patients with a condition at a specific point in time

d. The number of patients who test negative and don't have the condition

e. The number of patients who test positive and have the condition

42. You are designing a study to assess patients' perception of pain during insertion of a progestogen-only contraceptive implant. You ask patients to rate their pain from 1 to 10 (1= no pain, 10= extreme pain).

How would you describe this type of data?

- **a.** Ordinal
- **b.** Nominal
- **c.** Binary
- **d.** Ratio
- **e.** Interval

43. A 23-year-old woman presents complaining of lower abdominal pain. She has noticed an increase in her vaginal discharge over the last few weeks and describes it as strong smelling. On vaginal examination, her vulva and vagina look normal; her cervix looks erythematous – 'strawberry cervix'.

What is the most likely cause for her symptoms?

- **a.** Bacterium *Streptococcus agalactiae*
- **b.** Bacterial vaginosis
- **c.** *Trichomonas vaginalis*
- **d.** *Candida albicans*
- **e.** *Chlamydia trachomatis*

44. You are reviewing results and find a positive result for bacterial vaginosis. The patient is 16 weeks pregnant with her second pregnancy, having had a previous vaginal delivery at 32 weeks.

What is the most appropriate treatment for this patient?

- **a.** Metronidazole 400mg twice daily for 5–7 days
- **b.** Intravaginal clindamycin 1% once daily for 7 days
- **c.** No treatment required as patient asymptomatic
- **d.** Metronidazole 1.5g single dose
- **e.** Azithromycin 1g orally in a single dose

45. A 42-year-old woman is complaining of vulval itching and soreness. On examination, the vulva is red and inflamed with a small fissure. She also has lesions on the tops of her thighs, and you also notice a thick vaginal discharge at the introitus.

What is the most likely cause for her symptoms?

a. Lichen sclerosus

b. Allergic reaction

c. Dermatitis

d. *Candida albicans*

e. *Chlamydia trachomatis*

46. An 18-year-old woman presents complaining of lower abdominal pain and intermenstrual bleeding. On examination, she has lower abdominal tenderness, cervical excitation and green discharge. You suspect she might have pelvic inflammatory disease. Her observations are normal.

What is the most appropriate treatment?

a. Stat dose of intramuscular ceftriaxone and azithromycin

b. Stat dose of intramuscular ceftriaxone, oral doxycycline and metronidazole for 14 days

c. Intravenous ceftriaxone and doxycycline for 7 days

d. Oral doxycycline and metronidazole for 7 days

e. Intravenous clindamycin and gentamicin for 7 days

47. A 32-year-old woman who is 32 weeks pregnant has been diagnosed with primary syphilis.

What is the most appropriate treatment?

a. Benzathine penicillin G 2.4MU IM as a single dose

b. Benzathine penicillin G 2.4MU IM on days 1 and 8

c. Benzathine penicillin G 2.4 MU IM weekly on days 1, 8 and 15

d. Ceftriaxone 2g IM

e. Azithromycin 2g IM

48. Prior to surgical abortion, cervical preparation may be considered. After what gestation is it recommended that cervical preparation should be used?

a. 8 weeks

b. 10 weeks

c. 12 weeks

d. 14 weeks

e. 16 weeks

49. A 23-year-old woman presents to her GP with a positive pregnancy test; her last menstrual period was 6 weeks ago. She requests a termination of pregnancy. The GP refers her to the local termination service where she confirmed her decision.

How long should she expect between decision and procedure?

  a. 3 days

  b. 5 days

  c. 7 days

  d. 8 days

  e. 10 days

50. A 33-year-old woman presents complaining of heavy menstrual bleeding for the last 6 months. She is usually fit and well and isn't taking any medication at present. On examination, her abdomen is soft and non-tender, vaginal examination is normal.

What is the most appropriate investigation?

  a. Thyroid function tests

  b. Coagulation screen

  c. Serum ferritin

  d. Full blood count

  e. USS pelvis

51. A 48-year-old woman presents complaining of heavy menstrual bleeding. Her pelvic ultrasound scan reveals a 4cm posterior wall fibroid, distorting the endometrial cavity. A recent haemoglobin was 100g/L. She is not currently sexually active and would like to avoid surgery if possible.

What is the most appropriate treatment option for this patient?

  a. Levonorgestrel-containing intrauterine system (LNG-IUS)

  b. Uterine artery embolisation

  c. Hysterectomy

  d. Ulipristal acetate

  e. Tranexamic acid

52. A 53-year-old woman with a BMI of 46 attended clinic complaining of postmenopausal bleeding. She has an endometrial biopsy which shows endometrial hyperplasia without atypia.

What is the most appropriate management option for her?

a. Total laparoscopic hysterectomy

b. Total abdominal hysterectomy

c. Oral progestogen

d. LNG-IUS Mirena

e. Total laparoscopic hysterectomy with conservation of ovaries

53. A 49-year-old woman with a BMI of 38 has endometrial hyperplasia without atypia. She is being managed with LNG-IUS. You discuss follow-up with her.

What is the most appropriate follow-up for this patient?

a. Two negative endometrial biopsies 3 months apart then discharge

b. Two negative endometrial biopsies 6 months apart then discharge

c. Endometrial biopsy with two negative endometrial biopsies 6 months apart then yearly

d. Yearly USS for endometrial thickness

e. Yearly USS for endometrial thickness and yearly endometrial biopsy

54. Outpatient hysteroscopy has become an efficient way of investigating abnormal uterine bleeding. What is the most appropriate analgesia recommended for the procedure?

a. Co-codamol 1 hour prior to procedure

b. Paracetamol 1 hour prior to procedure

c. Diclofenac 1 hour prior to procedure

d. PR diclofenac during procedure

e. Conscious sedation

55. A 24-year-old woman has a pelvic USS to locate her intrauterine contraceptive device as the threads were not seen on vaginal examination. USS pelvis: 4cm simple left ovarian cyst, Cu-IUD correctly placed.

What is the most appropriate management for this patient's ovarian cyst?

a. No further management required

b. Repeat USS in 4 months

c. Repeat USS in 6 months

d. Repeat USS in 12 months

e. CA125

56. A 67-year-old woman attends complaining of vulval itching. On examination, you notice thinning of the skin and loss of pigmentation around the introitus. You take a vulval biopsy. The histology report shows: *epidermal thinning, hyperkeratosis, homogenised collagen below the dermo-epidermal junction with lymphocytic infiltrate.*

What is the most likely diagnosis?

a. Paget disease

b. Lichen sclerosus

c. Psoriasis

d. Lichen planus

e. Vulval intraepithelial neoplasia

57. Patients diagnosed with lichen sclerosus are advised to report any vulval changes early and return for annual review.

What is the risk of squamous cell carcinoma in a patient with lichen sclerosus?

a. <1%

b. 2–3%

c. 4%

d. <5%

e. 10%

58. A 36-year-old lady complains of vulval itching and burning. You examine her to find well defined, smooth erythematous lesions with sharp outlines on either side of the vulva, another lesion on the top of her thigh; on speculum examination, her vagina is not affected.

What is the most likely diagnosis?

a. Psoriasis

b. Lichen planus

c. Herpes simplex

d. Lichen simplex

e. Lichen sclerosus

59. Which of the following is not one of the five principal steps in an audit cycle?

   a. Selection of a topic

   b. Identification of an appropriate standard

   c. Implementation of changes to improve care

   d. Data collection for second time to determine if care has improved

   e. Create new knowledge to determine best practice

60. A 23-year-old woman had surgical evacuation of products of conception for a presumed molar pregnancy. She is awaiting histology results. She asks you what contraception she can use as this was an unplanned pregnancy while she was using the progestogen-only pill.

What is the most appropriate option?

   a. Combined hormonal contraceptive pill

   b. Cu-IUD

   c. LNG-IUS

   d. Progestogen implant

   e. Progestogen-only pill

Answers to practice paper 1 SBA questions

1. Correct response – C

   Explanation – emergency contraception providers should advise women using enzyme-inducing drugs that the effectiveness of UPA-EC and LNG-EC could be reduced. Women using enzyme-inducing drugs should be offered Cu-IUD. A 3mg dose of LNG can be considered but women should be informed that the effectiveness is unknown. Double dose of UPA-EC is not recommended.

   Reference – FSRH, *Emergency contraception*. March 2017 (updated May 2017).

2. Correct response – E

   Explanation – the risk of perforation with IUC is up to 2 in 1000 insertions and is approximately six-fold higher in breastfeeding women.

   Reference – FSRH, *Intrauterine contraception*. April 2015 (updated October 2015).

3. Correct response – B

   Explanation – there is no evidence as to the most appropriate treatment option for women with unscheduled bleeding with LNG-IUS. For women with unscheduled bleeding who wish to continue with the LNG-IUS, and are medically eligible, a combined oral contraceptive could be tried for up to 3 months.

   References – FSRH, *Intrauterine contraception*. April 2015 (updated October 2015).

4. Correct response – C

   Explanation – the SPC advises that the implant should be inserted 8–10cm up the arm from the medial epicondyle. Because of natural variation in arm lengths the guideline development group agreed that 8–10cm is not always the ideal distance and that as a general guide the insertion site should be one-third of the way up the arm from the elbow.

   Reference – FSRH, *Progestogen-only implants*. February 2014.

5. Correct response – B

   Explanation – the FSRH supports extended use of LNG-IUS 52mg (Mirena) for contraception until the age of 55 if inserted at age 45 or above, provided it is not being used as a progestogen component of hormone replacement therapy (HRT) for endometrial protection.

   Reference – FSRH, *Contraception for women aged over 40 years*. August 2017.

6. Correct answer – E

   Explanation – for women using progestogen-only contraception, the advice from the FSRH is to continue until age 55. Or check FSH levels – if FSH >30IU/L she can stop using contraception in 1 year.

   Reference – FSRH, *Contraception for women aged over 40 years*. August 2017.

7. Correct response – C

   Explanation – use expectant management for 7–14 days as the first line management strategy for women with a confirmed diagnosis of miscarriage.

   Reference – NICE, *Ectopic pregnancy and miscarriage: diagnosis and initial management*. CG154, December 2012.

8. Correct response – E

   Explanation – surgical management is indicated as the hCG is >5000IU/L, she has pain and the adnexal mass is 35mm. When surgical treatment is indicated for women with an ectopic pregnancy, it should be performed laparoscopically whenever possible, taking into account the condition of the woman.

   Reference – NICE, *Ectopic pregnancy and miscarriage: diagnosis and initial management*. CG154, December 2012.

9. Correct response – D

   Explanation – age-related risk of miscarriage at 30–34 is 15%.

   Reference – RCOG, *The investigation and treatment of couples with recurrent first-trimester and second trimester miscarriage*. GTG17, April 2011.

10. Correct response – D

    Explanation – presentation of a molar pregnancy can include abdominal distension due to a theca lutein cyst.

    Reference – RCOG, *The management of gestational trophoblastic disease*. GTG38, February 2010.

11. Correct response – C

    Explanation – if the hCG has reverted to normal within 56 days of the pregnancy event, follow-up will be for 6 months from the date of the uterine evacuation.

    Reference – RCOG, *The management of gestational trophoblastic disease*. GTG38, February 2010.

12. Correct response – E

Explanation – two moderate and one high risk factor are indications for aspirin from 12 weeks to reduce the risk of pre-eclampsia.

Reference – NICE, *Hypertension in pregnancy: diagnosis and management.* CG107, updated January 2011.

13. Correct response – D

Explanation – previous pre-eclampsia requiring delivery before 34 weeks has a 25% recurrence rate.

Reference – NICE, *Hypertension in pregnancy: diagnosis and management.* CG107, updated January 2011.

14. Correct response – B

Explanation – women with a primary lesion in the third trimester have a 41% risk of transmission, therefore prophylactic aciclovir and caesarean section is recommended.

Reference – RCOG and BASHH, *Management of genital herpes in pregnancy.* 2014.

15. Correct response – C

Reference – Bennett and Williamson, *Basic Sciences in Obstetrics and Gynaecology. A textbook for MRCOG Part 1, 4e.* 2010.

16. Correct response – D

Explanation – rhesus-negative women with a potentially sensitising event after 20 weeks of gestation, a minimum of 500IU anti-D Ig within 72 hours and test for foetal maternal haemorrhage.

Reference – Qureshi, Massey, Kirwan *et al.* BCSH guideline for the use of anti-D immunoglobulin for the prevention of haemolytic disease of the fetus and newborn. *Transfusion Medicine,* 2014;24:8.

17. Correct response – C

Explanation – women known to have group B streptococcus should be treated with intrapartum IV benzylpenicillin.

Reference – RCOG, *Group B streptococcal disease, early onset.* GTG36, 2017.

18. Correct response – B

Explanation – lacerations, one to two babies in every 100 (common).

Reference – RCOG, *Caesarean section Consent Advice* No. 7, October 2009.

19. Correct answer – E

Explanation – postpartum psychosis presents with delusions and hallucinations, and patients can appear confused and bewildered. Postpartum psychosis is a medical emergency. They should be cared for in a mother and baby unit.

Reference – NIC, *Antenatal and postnatal mental health: clinical management and service guideline.* August 2017.

20. Correct response – B

Explanation – offer vaginal oestrogen to women with urogenital atrophy (including those on systemic HRT) and continue treatment for as long as needed to relieve symptoms.

Reference – NICE, *Menopause diagnosis and management.* NG23, 2015.

21. Correct response – B

Explanation – menopause is defined as having occurred when a woman has not had a period for 12 consecutive months (for women reaching menopause naturally).

Reference – NICE, *Menopause diagnosis and management.* NG23, 2015.

22. Correct response – D

Reference – Otify, Fuller, Ross, *et al.* Endometrial pathology in the postmenopausal woman – an evidence based approach to management. *TOG,* 2015;17:29.

23. Correct response – D

Explanation – first line management of PMS includes exercise, CBT, vitamin B6, combined new generation pill, continuous or luteal phase low dose SSRI, e.g. citalopram. The COC in this case is UKMEC score of 3 so best avoided first line.

Reference – RCOG, *Management of premenstrual syndrome.* GTG48, February 2017.

24. Correct response – A

Explanation – when treating women with PMS, drospirenone-containing COCs may represent effective treatment for PMS and should be considered as a first line pharmaceutical intervention.

Reference – RCOG, *Management of premenstrual syndrome.* GTG48, February 2017.

25. Correct response – D

Explanation – when clinically reviewing women for PMS, symptoms should be recorded prospectively, over two cycles, using a symptoms diary, as retrospective recall of symptoms is unreliable.

Reference – RCOG, *Management of premenstrual syndrome.* GTG48, February 2017.

26. Correct response – E

Explanation – POI should be based on a combination of oligomenorrhoea/amenorrhoea associated with elevated levels of gonadotropins on at least two occasions 4–6 weeks apart.

Reference – NICE, *Menopause: diagnosis and management*. NG23, November 2015.

27. Correct response – C

Explanation – this patient has the classic symptoms of PCOS, menstrual disturbance and obesity, her bloods results show a 3:1 LH:FSH ratio often seen with PCOS. Also meets the Rotterdam criteria for diagnosis of PCOS.

Reference – Balen. Polycystic ovary syndrome. *TOG*, 2017;19:119.

28. Correct response – D

Explanation – women with hydrosalpinges should be offered salpingectomies, preferably by laparoscopy before IVF treatment as this improves the chance of live birth.

Reference – NICE, *Fertility problems*. QS73, October 2014.

29. Correct response – B

Explanation – women who are not known to have co-morbidities (such as pelvic inflammatory disease, previous ectopic or endometriosis) should be offered hysterosalpingography to screen for tubal occlusion.

Reference – NICE, *Fertility problems*. QS73, October 2014.

30. Correct response – B

Explanation – he is likely to be taking exogenous hormones which is having a negative feedback on his FSH and LH production.

31. Correct response – D

Explanation – measure post-void residual volume by bladder scan or catheterisation in women with symptoms suggestive of voiding dysfunction or recurrent UTIs.
Reference – NICE, *Urinary incontinence in women: management*. CG171, September 2013 (updated November 2015).

32. Correct response – D

Explanation – use bladder diaries in the initial assessment of women with urinary incontinence.

Reference – NICE, *Urinary incontinence in women: management*. CG171, September 2013 (updated November 2015).

33. Correct response – B

Explanation – offer a trial of pelvic floor muscle training of at least 3 months' duration as first line treatment to women with stress incontinence.

Reference – NICE, *Urinary incontinence in women: management.* CG171, September 2013 (updated November 2015).

34. Correct response – D

Explanation – HPV is a double-stranded DNA virus containing only eight genes.

Reference – StratOG.net: https://stratog.rcog.org.uk

35. Correct response – E

Explanation – atrophic endometritis and vaginitis is the most common cause of postmenopausal bleeding, accounting for up to 60–80%.

Reference – Otify, Fuller, Ross, *et al.* Endometrial pathology in the postmenopausal woman – an evidence based approach to management. *TOG*, 2015;17:29.

36. Correct answer – B

Explanation – endometrial polyps typically appear as hyperechoic lesions with regular contours in the uterine cavity surrounded by a thin hyperechoic halo.

Reference – Otify, Fuller, Ross, *et al.* Endometrial pathology in the postmenopausal woman – an evidence based approach to management. *TOG*, 2015;17:29.

37. Correct answer – B

Reference – Otify, Fuller, Ross, *et al.* Endometrial pathology in the postmenopausal woman – an evidence based approach to management. *TOG*, 2015;17:29.

38. Correct response – E

Explanation – a paired *t*-test compares an outcome on a single sample before and after an intervention.

Reference – Harris and Taylor, *Medical Statistics Made Easy, 3e.* 2014.

39. Correct response – D

Explanation – an unpaired *t*-test compares the means of two independent groups.

Reference – Harris and Taylor, *Medical Statistics Made Easy, 3e.* 2014.

40. Correct response – E

Reference – International Epidemiological Association (IEA). *Good epidemiological practice: IEA guidelines for proper conduct in epidemiologic research.* 2007.

41. Correct response – E

Explanation – the positive predictive value is the chance that a patient that tested positive has the condition.

Reference – Harris and Taylor, *Medical Statistics Made Easy, 3e*. 2014.

42. Correct response – A

Explanation – qualitative is used to describe characteristics. Ordinal data is a type of qualitative data that refers to quantities that have a natural ordering, i.e. pain scale.

43. Correct response – C

Explanation – *Trichomonas vaginalis* is a flagellated protozoan. Classic signs and symptoms include a strawberry cervix and foul-smelling discharge.

Reference – BASHH, *United Kingdom National guideline on the management of Trichomonas vaginalis.* 2014.

44. Correct response – A

Explanation – recommended regime is metronidazole 400mg twice daily for 5–7 days. There is insufficient evidence to recommend routine treatment of symptomatic pregnant women who attend a GU clinic and are found to have BV. Women with additional risk factors for preterm birth may benefit from treatment before 20 weeks.

Reference – BASHH, *United Kingdom National guideline for the management of bacterial vaginosis.* 2012.

45. Correct response – D

Explanation – vulvovaginal candidiasis usually presents with an itchy burning sensation. There can often be signs of erythema, fissuring, 'curd'-like discharge, oedema and satellite lesion.

Reference – BASHH, *United Kingdom National guideline for the management of vulvovaginal candidiasis.* 2007.

46. Correct response – B

Explanation – it is likely that delaying treatment increases the risk of long-term sequelae such as ectopic pregnancy. Outpatient management regimes include: IM ceftriaxone 500mg single dose followed by oral doxycycline 100mg twice daily plus metronidazole 400mg twice daily for 14 days.

Reference – BASHH, *United Kingdom National guideline for the management of pelvic inflammatory disease.* 2011.

47. Correct response – B

Explanation – in the third trimester (from 28 weeks) benzathine penicillin G 2.4MU IM on days 1 and 8.

Reference – BASHH, *United Kingdom National guideline for the management of syphilis*. 2015.

48. Correct response – D

Explanation – cervical preparation should be used for all women with a gestational age over 14 weeks.

Reference – RCOG, *Best practice in comprehensive abortion care.* Best practice paper No. 2, June 2015.

49. Correct response – B

Explanation – services should offer women the abortion procedure within 5 working days of the decision to proceed.

Reference – RCOG, *The care of women requesting induced abortion*. Evidence-based clinical guideline No. 7, November 2011.

50. Correct response – D

Explanation – a full blood count should be carried out on all women with heavy menstrual bleeding. Imaging is indicated if the uterus is palpable abdominally, vaginal examination reveals a pelvic mass of uncertain origin or pharmaceutical treatment fails.

Reference – NICE, *Heavy menstrual bleeding: assessment and management*. CG44, January 2007 (updated August 2016).

51. Correct response – D

Explanation – offer ulipristal acetate 5mg (up to 4 courses) to women with heavy menstrual bleeding and fibroids of 3cm or more in diameter and haemoglobin level of 102g/L or below.

Reference – NICE, *Heavy menstrual bleeding: assessment and management*. CG44, January 2007 (updated August 2016).

52. Correct response – D

Explanation – first line treatment for endometrial hyperplasia without atypia is LNG-IUS (Mirena).

Reference – RCOG, *Management of endometrial hyperplasia*. GTG67, February 2016.

53. Correct response – C

Explanation – in women at higher risk of relapse (i.e. BMI >35), 6-monthly endometrial biopsies, once two consecutive negative biopsies have been obtained; long-term follow-up should be considered with annual endometrial biopsies.

Reference – RCOG, *Management of endometrial hyperplasia*. GTG67, February 2016.

54. Correct answer – C

Explanation – NSAIDs 1 hour before their scheduled outpatient hysteroscopy appointment aims to reduce pain in the immediate postoperative period.

Reference – RCOG, *Best practice in outpatient hysteroscopy*. GTG59, March 2011.

55. Correct response – A

Explanation – women with small simple cysts (<50mm in diameter) generally do not require follow-up.

Reference – RCOG, *Management of suspected ovarian masses in premenopausal women*. GTG62, November 2011.

56. Correct response – B

Explanation – lichen sclerosus can present with itching and white atrophic areas affecting the vulva; changes can often be seen in a 'figure of 8' distribution.

Reference – BASHH, *United Kingdom National guideline for the management of vulval conditions*. 2014.

57. Correct response – D

Explanation – development of squamous cell carcinoma (actual risk <5%).

Reference – BASHH, *United Kingdom National guideline for the management of vulval conditions*. 2014.

58. Correct response – A

Explanation – symptoms of psoriasis include itching, soreness and burning. The lesions are often well demarcated brightly erythematous plaques, often symmetrical. They can have lesions on other areas such as upper thighs.

Reference – BASHH, *United Kingdom National guideline for the management of vulval conditions*. 2014.

59. Correct response – E

Explanation – audit ensures that the right thing is done properly.

Reference – RCOG, *Audit*. Clinical governance advice No. 5, October 2003.

60. Correct response – D

Explanation – most methods of contraception can be safely used after treatment for gestational trophoblastic disease and can be started immediately after uterine evacuation, with the exception of intrauterine contraception. This patient would benefit from the progestogen implant in view of her non-compliance with oral contraceptives.

Reference – FSRH, *Contraception after pregnancy*. January 2017.

Practice paper 2: SBA questions

1. Long-acting reversible contraceptives such as intrauterine devices are an effective form of contraception for many women.

   What is the risk of expulsion of intrauterine contraception?

   a. 1 in 10

   b. 1 in 20

   c. 1 in 50

   d. 1 in 100

   e. 1 in 1000

2. An asymptomatic 30-year-old patient with a copper intrauterine device (Cu-IUD) had a sexual health screen following an episode of unprotected sexual intercourse. *Actinomyces israelii* are identified on a high vaginal swab.

   What is the most appropriate management option?

   a. The IUD should be removed

   b. The patient should be treated with antibiotics for 6 weeks; the IUD can be left *in situ*

   c. No further action is required

   d. The patient should be treated with antibiotics for 6 weeks; the IUD should be removed

   e. The patient should be treated with cefalexin and metronidazole for 7 days; the IUD can be left *in situ*

3. A 26-year-old patient is struggling to remember to take her COC and she is requesting to have the progestogen-only implant inserted. She is allergic to latex therefore doesn't want to have to take additional precautions when she changes her method of contraception.

   When is the best time for her to switch contraceptives?

   a. Day 1–7 of hormone-free period

   b. Week 1 following hormone-free interval

   c. Week 2–3 of pill-taking period

   d. Day 1–5 of hormone-free period

   e. Day 1–3 of hormone-free period

4. What is the primary mode of action of the progestogen-only contraceptive implant?

Select the single best answer.

a. Prevents ovulation

b. Prevents fertilisation

c. Delays ovulation

d. Vaginal atrophy

e. Prevents implantation

5. A 42-year-old patient attends for contraceptive advice. She has a BMI of 25 and is a non-smoker with no medical or surgical history.

Which one of the following contraceptive options is the least appropriate?

a. Combined hormonal contraceptive with a low dose of ethinylestradiol

b. Progestogen-only pill

c. Progestogen-only injection

d. LNG-IUS 52mg

e. Progestogen-only implant

6. A 23-year-old woman attends the early pregnancy assessment unit complaining of vaginal bleeding and pelvic pain. On assessment, she is haemodynamically stable with minimal bleeding. Her last menstrual period was approximately 6 weeks ago.

Transvaginal ultrasound scan: *anteverted uterus with a gestational sac and foetal pole. Crown rump length = 7.0mm, no visible foetal heartbeat, both ovaries are seen with a small amount of free fluid behind the uterus.*

What is the most appropriate management plan?

a. Medical management of miscarriage

b. Repeat USS in 7 days

c. Repeat USS in 14 days

d. Surgical management of miscarriage

e. Check hCG and repeat in 48 hours

7. Misoprostol is used for the medical management of miscarriage.

What is the mechanism of action of misoprostol?

a. Synthetic prostaglandin E1 analogue

    b. Anti-progestogen

    c. Synthetic prostaglandin E2 analogue

    d. Serotonin receptor agonist

    e. Synthetic prostaglandin PGF2 alpha analogue

8. A 35-year-old woman is diagnosed with a missed miscarriage on USS at 8 weeks. She chooses to have medical management. This is her first pregnancy and she is blood group A RhD negative. What is the most appropriate management for this patient?

    a. Give 250IU anti-D rhesus prophylaxis

    b. Give 500IU anti-D rhesus prophylaxis

    c. Perform Kleihauer test to quantify feto-maternal haemorrhage and guide dose of anti-D the patient needs

    d. No need for anti-D rhesus prophylaxis

    e. Give 250IU anti-D now and a further 250IU in 72 hours

9. What percentage of couples trying to conceive are affected by recurrent miscarriage?

    a. 1%

    b. 2%

    c. 5%

    d. 7%

    e. 10%

10. A woman attends for a follow-up appointment after an EVAC for a molar pregnancy. She explains to you that this is her second molar pregnancy and she is concerned about this happening again in a future pregnancy.

What advice do you give her about the recurrence rate after two previous molar pregnancies?

    a. 1 in 10

    b. 1 in 20

    c. 1 in 30

    d. 1 in 45

    e. 1 in 55

11. A 35-year-old type 1 diabetic comes for pre-pregnancy counselling. She is using an insulin pump and her diabetes has been well controlled over the last few years. She is taking ramipril and simvastatin; her BMI is 30 and she is a smoker.

What would be the first step in her management?

a. Start 75mg of aspirin

b. Arrange a retinal and renal assessment

c. Commence 400mcg of folic acid

d. Medication review

e. Advice on diet and exercise

12. Pre-conceptual folic acid is recommended to reduce the risk of neural tube defects. High risk women including women with epilepsy require a higher dose of folic acid.

Which of the following is not an indication for high dose folic acid?

a. BMI >30

b. High blood pressure in previous pregnancy

c. Multiple pregnancy

d. Diabetes

e. Previous baby with a neural tube defect

13. Screening for diabetes in pregnancy is usually performed with a glucose tolerance test between 24 and 28 weeks.

Which one of the following is not an indication to screen for diabetes?

a. Previous gestational diabetes

b. Family history of first-degree relative with diabetes

c. Previous baby over 4.5kg

d. Age 35 or over

e. BMI 30 or over

14. A 33-year-old woman is seen 6 weeks postnatal for a debrief. She developed obstetric cholestasis at 35 weeks of gestation and was induced at 37 weeks. She wants to know the risk of having obstetric cholestasis again in a future pregnancy.

What is the risk of her developing obstetric cholestasis in a future pregnancy?

a. 10%

b. 20%

c. 30%

d. 40%

e. 90%

15. A 23-year-old woman attends antenatal clinic at 20+6 weeks. She has a history of genital herpes and is concerned about transmitting it to her baby.

What advice would you give her?

a. She will need delivery by caesarean section if lesions present when in labour

b. She can have a vaginal delivery

c. She will need delivery by caesarean section if she has a flare-up within 6 weeks of delivery

d. She will need to take aciclovir for 6 weeks prior to delivery if she wants a vaginal delivery

e. She can have a vaginal delivery with IV aciclovir during labour

16. In the foetal circulation which vessel shunts blood from the pulmonary artery to the descending aorta?

a. Foramen ovale

b. Ductus arteriosus

c. Ductus venosus

d. Ligamentum teres

e. Umbilical vein

17. During the third stage of labour it is recommended to give a uterotonic to decrease the risk of postpartum haemorrhage.

What is the most appropriate uterotonic to give following a normal vaginal delivery?

a. 5IU oxytocin IV

b. 5IU oxytocin IM

c. 10IU oxytocin IV

d. 10IU oxytocin IM

e. 500mcg ergometrine

18. A 23-year-old woman was diagnosed with a third-degree tear following a vaginal delivery. She was transferred to theatre for repair.

What is the risk of a woman acquiring a third-degree tear in her first pregnancy?

a. 2%

b. 4%

c. 6%

d. 8%

e. 10%

19. You see a 30-year-old woman with a BMI of 35 who is 4 weeks postnatal and wants to start using contraception. She had a normal vaginal delivery and is not breastfeeding.

What form of contraception should be avoided?

a. Combined hormonal contraception

b. Progestogen-only pill

c. Condoms

d. Intrauterine contraceptive

e. Progesterone-only implant

20. A 50-year-old patient with a BMI of 25 presents complaining of menopausal symptoms over the last 6 months which are interfering with her quality of life. She would like to use HRT to manage her symptoms. The patient is still having periods but they have been more irregular over the last 12 months.

What is the best management for this patient's symptoms?

a. Continuous combined HRT ideally started with the next period

b. Tibolone

c. Sequential HRT ideally started with the next period

d. Oestrogen-only HRT

e. Do not start HRT as she is not menopausal

21. A 46-year-old patient presents to your clinic; she hasn't had a period for 11 months. She is complaining of hot sweats at night, forgetfulness and low mood. You suspect that she is perimenopausal.

From the options below, what is the most appropriate investigation in this patient?

a. FSH

b. Oestradiol

c. Inhibin A

d. AMH

e. None of the above

22. What percentage of women experience premenstrual symptoms?

    a. 10%

    b. 20%

    c. 30%

    d. 40%

    e. 60%

23. A 24-year-old patient with a BMI of 22 presents complaining of anxiety and irritability. She describes these symptoms as cyclical, mainly occurring the week before her period. You suspect she may have premenstrual syndrome and give her a symptoms diary to complete.

What hormone is associated with premenstrual syndrome?

    a. Progesterone

    b. Oestrogen

    c. Follicle stimulating hormone

    d. Luteinising hormone

    e. Ethinylestradiol

24. Ovarian hyperstimulation syndrome (OHSS) is a complication of women undergoing fertility treatment.

What risk factor is associated with an increased risk of OHSS?

    a. High BMI

    b. Family history

    c. Multiple pregnancy

    d. High blood pressure

    e. Diabetes

25. A patient attends the gynaecology ward 2 weeks following an IVF cycle. Her symptoms include abdominal bloating, mild abdominal pain, nausea and vomiting. Transvaginal ultrasound: *9cm left ovary and a small amount of free fluid.* You diagnose ovarian hyperstimulation syndrome.

What is the best form of management for this patient?

a. Admit and manage as an inpatient

b. Reassure her and discharge

c. Manage as an outpatient and review in 2–3 days

d. Admit and administer IV fluids and anti-emetics

e. Admit and administer analgesia, anti-emetics and oral fluids

26. You are assessing a couple for infertility. After taking a history and arranging some initial investigations they ask you what could be the reason that they haven't conceived yet.

What is the most common cause of subfertility in the UK?

a. Unexplained

b. Disorders of ovulation

c. Maternal age

d. Male factors

e. Tubal damage

27. A 27-year-old woman with a BMI of 34 attends the fertility clinic. Her partner has had a normal semen analysis. Her investigations have confirmed PCOS.

What is the most appropriate next step in her management?

a. Clomifene citrate with metformin

b. Weight loss and review in 6 months

c. Clomifene

d. IVF

e. Metformin

28. A 29-year-old couple have been trying to conceive for 18 months. She has regular menstrual cycles and all her fertility investigations have been normal. His semen analysis was normal.

What is the next step in their management?

a. Continue trying, follow-up appointment in 6 months

b. Offer them a cycle of IVF

c. Clomifene citrate

d. Clomifene and metformin

e. Lifestyle advice and follow-up appointment in 6 months

29. Clomifene citrate is used as part of fertility treatment to induce ovulation.

What is the mechanism of action of clomifene?

a. Selective oestrogen receptor modulator

b. Gonadotrophin release hormone agonist

c. Dopamine receptor agonist

d. Synthetic gonadotrophin

e. Progesterone receptor modulator

30. A 60-year-old woman is complaining of urinary frequency. She has tried conservative measures but she hasn't seen any benefit so she comes to discuss pharmacological treatment. She is usually well and has a normal blood pressure.

What is the most appropriate first line treatment?

a. Imipramine

b. Mirabegron

c. Tolterodine

d. Duloxetine

e. Desmopressin

31. A 58-year-old woman attends clinic complaining of urinary urgency and frequency. She has had two urinary tract infections this year. On examination, her abdomen is soft and non-tender, she has a grade 1 uterine prolapse and a dry and erythematous vaginal mucosa.

What is the most appropriate treatment for this patient's symptoms?

a. Oxybutynin

b. Vaginal oestrogen therapy

c. Systemic hormone replacement therapy

d. Duloxetine

e. Steroid cream

32. A 53-year-old postmenopausal woman presents complaining of altered bowel habits over the last few months. She describes feeling full after a small amount of food and often feels bloated.

What is the most appropriate investigation to perform?

- **a.** USS abdomen/pelvis
- **b.** CT abdomen/pelvis
- **c.** CA125
- **d.** Urine sample
- **e.** Colonoscopy

33. Ovarian cancer often presents at an advanced stage.

Which one of the following is a risk factor for ovarian cancer?

- **a.** Breastfeeding
- **b.** Tubal ligation
- **c.** Hysterectomy
- **d.** Combined oral contraceptive pill
- **e.** Nulliparity

34. A 68-year-old woman presents with a 6 month history of acid reflux and bloating. Her risk of malignancy index is >700. A recent CT scan shows a 5×5cm right-sided pelvic mass, free fluid, omental and peritoneal deposits and parenchymal liver metastasis.

What is the most appropriate management?

- **a.** Referral to oncologist for further treatment
- **b.** Palliative care
- **c.** Omental biopsy and paracentesis
- **d.** Total abdominal hysterectomy, bilateral salpingo-oophorectomy, omentectomy
- **e.** Smear

35. A 32-year-old woman with HIV received a letter with her smear results. She has low grade dyskaryosis, high grade HPV negative.

What is the most appropriate follow-up for the patient?

- **a.** Refer to colposcopy
- **b.** Repeat smear in 6 months
- **c.** Repeat smear in 1 year

d. Repeat smear in 3 years

e. Repeat smear in 5 years

36. A 35-year-old woman was seen in colposcopy following a smear result of high grade dyskaryosis. Colposcopy reveals changes consistent with CIN2 which was treated.

What is the most appropriate follow-up for this patient?

a. Test of cure in 3 months

b. Test of cure in 6 months

c. Colposcopy in 6 months

d. Colposcopy in 12 months

e. Routine 3 yearly recall

37. A 48-year-old has a total laparoscopic hysterectomy due to failed medical management of heavy menstrual bleeding. You review the histology to find that there was CIN in the specimen which was completely excised.

What is the most appropriate follow-up for this patient?

a. No follow-up required

b. Vault smear in 6 months

c. Vault smear in 6 and 18 months

d. Vault smear in 6, 12 and 24 months

e. Vault smear in 6 and 12 months, then yearly for 9 years

38. What is the risk of progression from endometrial hyperplasia with atypia to endometrial cancer if left untreated?

a. 10%

b. 15%

c. 23%

d. 30%

e. 35%

39. Standard deviation is used to interpret results in research studies.

Which one of the following defines standard deviation?

a. Provides information on how much the data varies around the mean

b. Provides information on how much the data varies around the median

    c. Describes the most frequently occurring event

    d. Describes the effect of treatment of a risk factor

    e. Describes how significant a result is

40. You are designing a study to look at the incidence of ovarian tumours in women taking the COC and women not taking the COC. What type of study would you use?

    a. Case control

    b. Cohort

    c. Randomised control trial

    d. Cross-sectional

    e. Double-blind randomised control trial

41. You are designing a study to look at the prevalence of chlamydia in patients under 25. What study design would you use?

    a. Case control

    b. Cohort

    c. Randomised control trial

    d. Cross-sectional

    e. Double-blind randomised control trial

42. Research data is divided into two groups, quantitative and qualitative.

Which one of the following is an example of quantitative data?

    a. Ordinal data

    b. Nominal data

    c. Binary data

    d. Ratio

    e. Variance data

43. You design a study to assess whether having a chlamydia infection affects future fertility. What is the most appropriate type of analytic test?

    a. Chi-squared

    b. Pearson's regression

    c. Mann–Whitney U

    d. Two sample (unpaired) t-test

    e. One sample (paired) t-test

44. A 23-year-old patient reports a thin white discharge. You take a vaginal swab to perform a wet mount, you see clue cells on microscopy and the vaginal pH is increased.

What is the most likely causative organism?

a. Bacterium *Streptococcus agalactiae*

b. Bacterial vaginosis

c. *Trichomonas vaginalis*

d. *Candida albicans*

e. *Chlamydia trachomatis*

45. What is the rate of mother-to-child transmission of HIV in the UK from women diagnosed with HIV?

a. 0.57%

b. 0.79%

c. 1%

d. 2%

e. 2.5%

46. A 24-year-old man reports having unprotected receptive anal sex with a man known to have HIV. You assess him to be high risk and therefore recommend post-exposure prophylaxis.

What treatment will you offer him?

a. Truvada and raltegravir for 28 days

b. Kaletra and darunavir for 28 days

c. Atazanavir and dolutegravir for 28 days

d. Truvada and Combivir for 28 days

e. Raltegravir and Kaletra for 28 days

47. A 28-year-old woman who is currently 37 weeks pregnant attends antenatal clinic to discuss mode of delivery. She is known to have HIV and has been taking combined antiretroviral therapy (ART). At 36+2 weeks her viral load was 40 HIV RNA copies/ml.

What best advice would you give her?

a. Recommend a vaginal delivery

b. Recommend a caesarean section

c. Aim for a vaginal delivery with an induction at 38 weeks

d. Recommend a vaginal delivery with an intrapartum zidovudine infusion

e. Recommend a caesarean section with a zidovudine infusion

48. A 26-year-old woman known to be HIV positive attends at 38+2 weeks with ruptured membranes. She is 8cm dilated. She is on ART, her last viral load was taken 2 weeks ago (85 HIV RNA copies/ml). She progresses quickly to have a normal vaginal delivery.

What is the most appropriate management for the baby?

a. Zidovudine monotherapy

b. Triple combination post-exposure prophylaxis within 4 hours of birth

c. Screen for HIV within 24 hours

d. Give *Pneumocystis* pneumonia prophylaxis

e. Encourage breastfeeding

49. A 26-year-old patient attends clinic for a termination of pregnancy. You perform a transvaginal ultrasound scan and find that she has a 6+3/40 intrauterine pregnancy; she decides to have a surgical termination of pregnancy.

What is the risk of uterine perforation?

a. 1 in 10

b. 1 in 100

c. 1 in 1000

d. 1 in 10 000

e. 1 in 100 000

50. An 18-year-old woman is referred from general practice for a medical termination for pregnancy. Her booking scan found her to be 19 weeks and 3 days.

After what gestation should feticide be performed to decrease the risk of live birth prior to medical abortion?

a. 18 weeks

b. 20 weeks

c. 20 weeks 5 days

d. 21 weeks 6 days

e. 22 weeks 6 days

51. When counselling a woman about the risk of termination of pregnancy there is a small risk of the need for further intervention to complete the procedure both medically and surgically.

What is the risk of further intervention following termination of pregnancy?

a. 1%

b. <5%

c. <7%

d. <10%

e. 15%

52. A 28-year-old nullip presents complaining of heavy periods despite having an LNG-IUS fitted 12 months ago and failed medical management. USS pelvis confirmed the LNG-IUS is positioned correctly and identifies a 5 × 5cm posterior wall fibroid. She would like to consider further treatment.

What is the most appropriate management option for her?

a. Laparoscopic hysterectomy with ovarian conservation

b. Total abdominal hysterectomy

c. Uterine artery ablation

d. Myomectomy

e. Endometrial ablation

53. Which of the following is not a risk factor for endometrial hyperplasia?

a. High BMI

b. Granulosa cell tumour

c. Tamoxifen

d. Oestrogen-only HRT

e. Fibroids

54. What size of hysteroscope is recommended for use in outpatient hysteroscopy?

a. 2.4mm with 2.8–3.3mm sheath

b. 2.5mm with 2.8–3.3mm sheath

c. 2.7mm with 3.0–3.5mm sheath

d. 2.9mm with 3.0–3.5mm sheath

e. 3.0mm with 3.3–3.5mm sheath

55. A 45-year-old patient with a long history of PCOS attends your clinic. She has had one menstrual period in the last year. She is not using any contraception or menopausal hormone therapy. You are concerned regarding her increased risk of endometrial cancer.

Which of the following options is the most appropriate initial management?

a. Arrange a pelvic USS; an ET <10mm is reassuring

b. Commence patient on medroxyprogesterone acetate BD for 7 days to induce a withdrawal bleed

c. Start her on the COC

d. Insert a Mirena

e. Arrange a pelvic USS; an ET <7mm is reassuring

56. The Rotterdam criteria are used to diagnose PCOS.

Which one of the following is part of the criteria?

a. Polycystic ovaries with over 8 follicles, anovulation/olio-ovulation, clinical/biochemical signs of hyperandrogenism

b. Polycystic ovaries with over 12 follicles, anovulation/olio-ovulation, clinical/biochemical signs of hyperandrogenism

c. Polycystic ovaries with over 8 follicles, anovulation/olio-ovulation, clinical/biochemical signs of high LH

d. Polycystic ovaries with over 8 follicles, anovulation/olio-ovulation, clinical/biochemical signs of hypertestosterone

e. Polycystic ovaries, anovulation/olio-ovulation, clinical/biochemical signs of hyperandrogenism

57. A 32-year-old woman has an abdominal USS to investigate recurrent urinary tract infections. The ultrasound reveals a 7cm, simple right ovarian cyst, normal anteverted uterus, normal left ovary.

What is the most appropriate management for this patient's ovarian cyst?

a. No further management required

b. Repeat USS in 4 months

c. Repeat USS in 6 months

d. Repeat USS in 12 months

e. CA125

58. A 57-year-old woman attends complaining of dyspareunia. You examine her and notice some pallor, labial fusion and her introitus is slightly narrowed.

What is the most likely diagnosis?

a. Lichen sclerosus

b. Atrophic vaginitis

c. Lichen planus

d. Vulval eczema

e. Lichen simplex

59. A 59-year-old woman attends complaining of dyspareunia. You examine her and notice some pallor, labial fusion and her introitus is slightly narrowed.

What is the most appropriate treatment?

a. Topical oestrogen

b. Clobetasol propionate

c. Topical calcineurin inhibitor

d. Hydrocortisone ointment

e. Emollient soap

60. Vulval intraepithelial neoplasia is a skin condition which may become cancerous if left untreated. The commonest cause of the usual VIN is human papillomavirus.

What is the commonest strain of HPV that causes VIN?

a. HPV 6

b. HPV 11

c. HPV 13

d. HPV 16

e. HPV 33

Answers to practice paper 2 SBA questions

1. Correct response – B

   Explanation – the risk of expulsion with IUC is around 1 in 20 and is most common in the first year of use, particularly in the first 3 months.

   Reference – FSRH, *Intrauterine contraception*. April 2015 (updated October 2015).

2. Correct response – C

   Explanation – there is no need to remove an IUD in asymptomatic women with ALOs.

   Reference – FSRH, *Intrauterine contraception*. April 2015 (updated October 2015).

3. Correct response – C

   Explanation – either day 1 of hormone-free/pill-free period or week 2–3. No additional contraceptive precautions or emergency contraception required as long as the patient has taken hormonally active pills for 7 consecutive days. There is evidence to suggest this is sufficient to prevent ovulation.

   Reference – FSRH, *Progestogen-only implants*. February 2014.

4. Correct response – A

   Explanation – the primary mode of action is to prevent ovulation. Implants also prevent sperm penetration by altering the cervical mucus and possibly preventing implantation by thinning the endometrium.

   Reference – FSRH, *Progestogen-only implants*. February 2014.

5. Correct answer – C

   Explanation – depot medroxyprogesterone acetate is associated with an initial loss in bone density due to the hypoestrogenic effects.

   Reference – FSRH, *Contraception for women aged over 40 years*. August 2017.

6. Correct response – B

   Explanation – if the CRL is 7.0mm or more with a transvaginal ultrasound scan and there is no visible heartbeat, either seek a second opinion and/or perform a second scan a minimum of 7 days after the first before making diagnosis of a failed pregnancy.

   Reference – NICE, *Ectopic pregnancy and miscarriage: diagnosis and initial management*. CG154, December 2012.

7. Correct response – A

Explanation – misoprostol is a synthetic prostaglandin E1 analogue.

8. Correct response – D

Explanation – do not offer anti-D rhesus prophylaxis to women who receive solely medical management of an ectopic or miscarriage, have a threatened or complete miscarriage, or have a pregnancy of unknown location. Offer anti-D rhesus prophylaxis at a dose of 250IU (50mcg) to all rhesus-negative women who have a surgical procedure to manage an ectopic pregnancy or a miscarriage.

Reference – NICE, *Ectopic pregnancy and miscarriage: diagnosis and initial management*. CG154, December 2012.

9. Correct response – A

Explanation – a diagnosis of recurrent miscarriage is made following the loss of three or more consecutive pregnancies; it affects 1% of couples trying to conceive.

Reference – RCOG, *The investigation and treatment of couples with recurrent first trimester and second trimester miscarriage*. GTG17, April 2011.

10. Correct response – A

Explanation – women who have had one previous molar pregnancy have a 1 in 55 risk of recurrence, while those who have had two have a 1 in 10 risk of recurrence.

Reference – Savage. Molar pregnancy. *TOG*, 2008;10:308.

11. Correct response – D

Explanation – ramipril and simvastatin are contraindicated in pregnancy. She will need high dose folic acid (5mg). Aspirin and diet/exercise advice are appropriate answers but a medication review is the most appropriate at this stage.

Reference – NICE, *Diabetes in pregnancy: management from preconception to the postnatal period*. NG53, February 2015.

12. Correct response – B

Explanation – high dose folic acid (5mg) should be given to women at higher risk of neural tube defects; these include personal or family history of neural tube defect, BMI >30 and other medical conditions such as epilepsy and thalassaemia.

Reference – NICE, *Maternal and child nutrition*. PH11, updated November 2014.

13. Correct response – D

Explanation – risk factors for diabetes include: BMI >30, previous macrosomic baby, previous gestational diabetes, family history of diabetes, minority ethnic family origin with high prevalence of diabetes.

Reference – NICE, *Diabetes in pregnancy: management from preconception to the postnatal period*. NG53, February 2015.

14. Correct response – E

Explanation – obstetric cholestasis has a recurrence rate of up to 90%.

Reference – RCOG, *Obstetric cholestasis*. GTG43, 2011.

15. Correct response – B

Explanation – recurrent genital herpes carries a very low transmission rate (0.3%) even if lesions are present during vaginal delivery.

Reference – RCOG and BASHH, *Management of genital herpes in pregnancy*. 2014.

16. Correct response – B

Reference – Bennett and Williamson, *Basic Sciences in Obstetrics and Gynaecology. A textbook for MRCOG Part 1*, 4e. 2010.

17. Correct response – D

Explanation – for women without risk of PPH delivering vaginally, oxytocin 10IU IM is the agent of choice for prophylaxis in the third stage.

Reference – RCOG, *Prevention and management of postpartum haemorrhage*. GTG52, December 2016.

18. Correct response – C

Explanation – the overall incidence of third-degree tears in the UK is 2.9% with an incidence of 6.1% in primiparae compared with 1.7% in multiparae.

Reference – RCOG, *The management of third and fourth degree perineal tears*. GTG29, June 2015.

19. Correct response – A

Explanation – all women should undergo a risk assessment for VTE postnatally. Women with risk factors should not use CHC within 6 weeks of childbirth. Risks for VTE include immobility, blood transfusion, BMI >30, postpartum haemorrhage, post-caesarean section, pre-eclampsia, smoking.

Reference – FSRH, *Contraception after pregnancy*. January 2017.

20. Correct response – C

Explanation – menopausal symptoms often start in the perimenopause. To avoid unnecessary investigation of unscheduled bleeds, perimenopausal women should be commenced on sequential HRT (this is continuous oestrogen with progestogen for 12–14 days per month).

Reference – Bakour and Williamson, Latest evidence on using hormone replacement therapy in menopause. *TOG*, 2015;17:20.

21. Correct response – E

Explanation – there is no need to use laboratory investigations in an otherwise healthy woman aged over 45 years with menopausal symptoms.

Reference – NICE, *Menopause diagnosis and management*. NG23, 2015.

22. Correct response – D

Reference – RCOG, *Management of premenstrual syndrome*. GTG48, February 2017.

23. Correct response – A

Explanation – in order to differentiate physiological menstrual symptoms from PMS it must be demonstrated that symptoms cause significant impairment to the individual during the luteal phase of the menstrual cycle.

Reference – RCOG, *Management of premenstrual syndrome*. GTG48, February 2017.

24. Correct answer – C

Explanation – risk factors include previous OHSS, PCOS, increased antral follicle count, high levels of anti-Müllerian hormone, multiple pregnancy.

Reference – RCOG, *The management of ovarian hyperstimulation syndrome*. GTG5, February 2016.

25. Correct answer – C

Explanation – this patient has mild to moderate OHSS. Mild, moderate and selected cases of severe OHSS can be managed as an outpatient.

Reference – RCOG, *The management of ovarian hyperstimulation syndrome*. GTG5, February 2016.

26. Correct response – D

Explanation – factors in the male causing infertility account for 30%, unexplained infertility 25%, ovulatory disorders 25%, tubal damage 20%, uterine or peritoneal disorders 10%.

Reference – NICE, *Fertility problems*. QS73, October 2014.

27. Correct response – B

Explanation – women with a BMI of 30 or over who are not ovulating should be informed that losing weight is likely to increase their chances of conception.

Reference – NICE, *Fertility problems*. QS73, October 2014.

28. Correct response – E

Explanation – offer IVF treatment to women with unexplained infertility who have not conceived after 2 years of regular unprotected sexual intercourse.

Reference – NICE, *Fertility problems*. QS73, October 2014.

29. Correct response – A

Explanation – clomifene is a selective oestrogen receptor modulator.

30. Correct response – C

Explanation – when considering pharmacological management of overactive or mixed urinary incontinence, offer either oxybutynin, tolterodine or darifenacin first before considering other pharmacological treatments such as mirabegron.

Reference – NICE, *Urinary incontinence in women: management*. CG171, September 2013 (updated November 2015).

31. Correct response – B

Explanation – offer intravaginal oestrogen for the treatment of overactive bladder symptoms in postmenopausal women with vaginal atrophy.

Reference – NICE, *Urinary incontinence in women: management*. CG171, September 2013 (updated November 2015).

32. Correct response – C

Explanation – carry out appropriate tests for ovarian cancer in any woman over 20 who has experienced symptoms within the last 12 months that suggest irritable bowel syndrome, because IBS rarely presents for the first time in women of this age.

Reference – NICE, *Ovarian cancer: the recognition and initial management of ovarian cancer*. April 2011 (developed for NICE by the National Collaborating Centre for Cancer).

33. Correct response – E

Reference – www.cancerresearchuk.org

34. Correct response – C

Explanation – this patient has advanced ovarian cancer; she is likely to be managed with cytotoxic chemotherapy. When offering chemotherapy to women with suspected advanced ovarian cancer, first obtain a confirmed tissue diagnosis by histology.

Reference – NICE, *Ovarian cancer: the recognition and initial management of ovarian cancer.* April 2011 (developed for NICE by the National Collaborating Centre for Cancer).

35. Correct response – C

Explanation – all HIV-positive women should have yearly smears.

Reference – NHS Cervical Screening Programme, *Colposcopy and programme management.* NHSCSP Publication number 20, March 2016.

36. Correct response – B

Explanation – CIN 1/2/3 treated, invite for 6 month test of cure.

Reference – NHS Cervical Screening Programme, *Colposcopy and programme management.* NHSCSP Publication number 20, March 2016.

37. Correct response – C

Explanation – CIN in specimen which is completely excised requires a vault smear in 6 and 18 months.

Reference – NHS Cervical Screening Programme, *Colposcopy and programme management.* NHSCSP Publication number 20, March 2016.

38. Correct answer – C

Reference – Otify, Fuller, Ross, *et al.* Endometrial pathology in the postmenopausal woman – an evidence based approach to management. *TOG*, 2015;17:29.

39. Correct response – A

Explanation – A standard deviation is used for data which are 'normally distributed', to provide information on how much data vary around their mean.

Reference – Harris and Taylor, *Medical Statistics Made Easy, 3e.* 2014.

40. Correct response – B

Explanation – a group with a common exposure followed to determine an outcome.

Reference – Harris and Taylor, *Medical Statistics Made Easy, 3e.* 2014.

41. Correct response – D

Explanation – cross-sectional study is a type of observational study that analyses data collected from a population at a specific point in time.

Reference – Harris and Taylor, *Medical Statistics Made Easy, 3e.* 2014.

42. Correct response – D

Explanation – quantitative data is data that can be measured numerically such as height, weight, blood pressure. Qualitative data is used to describe characteristics such as eye colour, pain scale. Ratio is a type of quantitative data.

43. Correct response – A

Explanation – the chi-squared test describes the association between two categorical variables.

Reference – Harris and Taylor, *Medical Statistics Made Easy, 3e.* 2014.

44. Correct response – B

Explanation – Amsel's criteria: at least three of the four criteria are present for the diagnosis to be confirmed, 1. Thin, white, homogeneous discharge; 2. Clue cells; 3. pH of vaginal fluid >4.5; 4. Release of a fishy odour on adding alkali (10% KOH).

Reference – BASHH, *United Kingdom National guideline for the management of bacterial vaginosis.* 2012.

45. Correct response – A

Explanation – in the UK the rate of HIV mother-to-child transmission from diagnosed women has dropped from 25.6% to 0.57%.

Reference – British HIV Association, Guideline for the management of HIV infection in pregnant women 2012 (2014 interim review). *HIV Medicine,* 2014;15(Suppl.4):1.

46. Correct response – A

Explanation – the first line regime for post-exposure prophylaxis following sexual exposure is Truvada and raltegravir for 28 days.

Reference – Cresswell, Waters, Briggs, *et al.* UK guideline for the use of HIV post-exposure prophylaxis following sexual exposure (2015). *International Journal of STD & AIDS,* 2016;27:713.

47. Correct response – A

Explanation – women taking cART should have a viral load performed at 36 weeks; if it is <50 HIV RNA copies/ml and there are no other obstetric contraindications she can aim for a vaginal delivery.

Reference – British HIV Association, Guideline for the management of HIV infection in pregnant women 2012 (2014 interim review). *HIV Medicine,* 2014;15(Suppl.4):1.

48. Correct response – B

Explanation – three-drug infant therapy is recommended for all circumstances where maternal viral load at 36 weeks of gestation is not <50 HIV RNA copies/ml.

Reference – British HIV Association, Guideline for the management of HIV infection in pregnant women 2012 (2014 interim review). *HIV Medicine,* 2014;15(Suppl.4):1.

49. Correct response – C

Explanation – uterine perforation: the risk is in the order of 1–4 in 1000 and is lower for early abortions and those performed by experienced clinicians.

Reference – RCOG, *The care of women requesting induced abortion*. EBCG7, November 2011.

50. Correct response – D

Explanation – feticide should be performed before medical abortion after 21 weeks and 6 days of gestation to ensure that there is no risk of live birth.

Reference – RCOG, *The care of women requesting induced abortion*. EBCG7, November 2011.

51. Correct response – B

Explanation – women should be informed that there is a small risk (usually less than 5%) of the need for further intervention, such as surgical intervention, following medical abortion or re-evacuation following surgical abortion.

Reference – RCOG, *The care of women requesting induced abortion*. EBCG7, November 2011.

52. Correct response – D

Explanation – she is young and hasn't had any children therefore her fertility needs to be preserved. NICE recommends myomectomy to retain fertility for fibroids over 3cm.

Reference – NICE, *Heavy menstrual bleeding: assessment and management*. CG44, January 2007 (updated August 2016).

53. Correct response – E

Explanation – oestrogen-only HRT, granulosa cell tumour (oestrogen-secreting tumour) and a high BMI are all related to high oestrogen levels; oestrogen stimulates growth of the endometrium which can lead to endometrial hyperplasia. Tamoxifen is a selective oestrogen receptor modulator most commonly used to treat oestrogen receptor positive breast cancer; however, it acts as a partial agonist on the endometrium and therefore can lead to endometrial hyperplasia.

Reference – RCOG, *Management of endometrial hyperplasia*. GTG,67, February 2016.

54. Correct response – C

Reference – RCOG, *Best practice in outpatient hysteroscopy*. GTG59, March 2011.

55. Correct response – E

Explanation – arrange an USS. It is important that these women have 3–4 bleeds per year. Transvaginal USS should be considered in the absence of withdrawal bleed or abnormal uterine bleeding. In PCOS an ET of <7mm is unlikely to be hyperplasia.

Reference – RCOG, *Long-term consequences of polycystic ovary syndrome*. GTG33, November 2014.

56. Correct response – B

Explanation – Rotterdam criteria 2003 includes: polycystic ovaries (either >12 follicles or ovarian volume over 10cm^3, oligo-ovulation or anovulation, clinical or biochemical signs of hyperandrogenism.

Reference – RCOG, *Long-term consequences of polycystic ovary syndrome*. GTG33, November 2014.

57. Correct response – D

Explanation – women with simple ovarian cysts of 50–70mm in diameter should have yearly USS follow-up.

Reference – RCOG, *Management of suspected ovarian masses in premenopausal women*. GTG62, November 2011.

58. Correct response – B

Explanation – offer vaginal oestrogen to women with urogenital atrophy (including those on systemic HRT) and continue treatment for as long as needed to relieve symptoms.

Reference – NICE, *Menopause diagnosis and management*. NG23, 2015.

59. Correct response – A

Explanation – offer vaginal oestrogen to women with urogenital atrophy (including those on systemic HRT) and continue treatment for as long as needed to relieve symptoms.

Reference – NICE, *Menopause diagnosis and management*. NG23, 2015.

60. Correct response – D

Explanation – in genitourinary clinics the most common aetiological agent is human papillomavirus; this is known as usual type and is mainly associated with HPV 16.

Reference – BASHH, *United Kingdom National guideline for the management of vulval conditions*. 2014.

Part
TWO

Introduction to MFSRH Part Two

Part Two of the MFSRH examination has three components including Critical Reading Questions (CRQ), Extended Matching Questions (EMQ) and an Objective Structured Clinical Examination (OSCE). The three parts of the exam take place on the same day once a year. Two years of clinical experience is recommended prior to taking this part of the exam. Candidates must pass the OSCE section of the exam and achieve a pass or borderline fail in the other two components, resulting in an overall pass.

The CRQ takes the form of a 90 minute written examination and is responsible for one-third of the overall marks. There are three questions with equal weighting. These will be composed of either part of an academic paper or a statistical diagram followed by questions. Answers should be provided as bullet points or in note form.

The EMQ is a 2 hour written paper with 80 questions designed to test clinical reasoning ability. This section of the exam is structured into four parts including theme, options, question and item.

The OSCE is designed to assess the candidate's ability to gather information, apply clinical skills, demonstrate patient-centred care and make evidence-based decisions. There are 10 active stations with each station lasting 12 minutes, including 3 minutes for reading.

To guide your revision, it is essential that you familiarise yourself with the 'Syllabus for MFSRH Part Two' which is in the 'MFSRH Part Two Handbook' found on the FSRH website (www.fsrh.org).

The curriculum modules covered by MFSRH Part two include:

- **Module 1:** Clinical skills
- **Module 2:** Contraception
- **Module 3:** Unplanned pregnancy and abortion care
- **Module 4:** Gynaecology (medical and surgical)
- **Module 5:** Speciality gynaecology (subfertility, gynaecological oncology, urogynaecology)
- **Module 6:** Pregnancy (antenatal, intrapartum, postnatal)
- **Module 7:** Menopause and premenstrual syndrome
- **Module 8:** Genitourinary medicine
- **Module 9:** Public health
- **Module 10:** Teaching, appraisal and assessment
- **Module 11:** Ethics and legal issues
- **Module 12:** Leadership, management and governance

- **Module 13:** Information technology, audit and research
- **Module 14:** Sexual assault
- **Module 15:** Sexual problems

The 'MFSRH Part Two Handbook' also has a reading list. This is an invaluable list of resources on which the questions in the examination are based.

Hints and tips for the Extended Matching Questions paper

The extended matching questions (EMQs) each have a theme and you will be given questions which will require you to be able to select the best answer from a list of between 6 and 10 options. You will find that the options may be quite similar, thus making it harder to 'guess' the answer and ensuring that these types of questions are a reliable method of assessing knowledge base.

1. Make a planner and divide your syllabus and what you need to read into manageable chunks – try to allocate a number of topics to your 'to do' list for each week and try to stick to your schedule. Tick off topics as you cover them.

2. Read to ensure a sound knowledge base! Try to do questions related to the topics you have read, as you go along.

3. Focus on your weak areas – the topics you want to avoid are the ones you should think of tackling first! This improves confidence and will help you stick to your schedule better.

4. Make notes – this can be helpful and it will help you cover salient points in the lead up to the exam.

5. Practise – practising as many questions as you can is crucial. Remember practice makes progress! Look at the reading list on the FSRH website for recommended EMQ revision books (and try all the EMQs which follow in this book of course!).

6. Discuss – some people find discussing a topic they have read with a study partner helpful. They may have read something which you haven't so make use of each other.

7. Time yourself – this will ensure you are exam ready. There are 80 questions in the exam so you should be able to pace yourself to get through those in the allocated time of 2 hours.

8. Approach each question independently and read it carefully – sometimes it may specify that the same answer may be used more than once.

9. Try to think what your answer would be to the question before you read the list of options.

10. Last but not least, believe in yourself. If you have done the required reading there is no reason that you shouldn't do well.

Extended Matching Questions

1–3. What is the most likely diagnosis?

    a. Labial adhesions

    b. Bartholin's cyst

    c. Imperforate hymen

    d. Transverse vaginal septum

    e. Endometriosis

    f. Gartner duct cyst

    g. Vaginal atresia

For each scenario described below, choose the SINGLE most likely diagnosis from the above list of options. Each option may be used once, more than once, or not at all.

1. A 14-year-old girl attends your clinic with her mother complaining of lower abdominal pain each month. She has normal breast development as well as pubic and axillary hair but has not yet started her periods. On vaginal inspection, you notice a bulging blue membrane.

2. A 10-month-old baby girl is brought to your clinic. Her mother is extremely anxious. She has noticed dribbling of urine even after changing her daughter's nappy and states "things don't look normal down below". On examination, you cannot clearly identify a vaginal opening.

3. A 22-year-old woman complains of a lump in her vulval area which has gradually increased in size. Although it is painless, it is now causing slight discomfort when she sits down. On examination you see a right-sided, unilateral swelling of 2cm involving the posterolateral aspect of the introitus.

4–6. Which is the most appropriate treatment option?

    a. Oxybutynin

    b. Duloxetine

    c. Desmopressin

    d. Total abdominal hysterectomy

    e. Tension-free vaginal tape

    f. Darifenacin

g. Anterior vaginal repair

h. Endometrial ablation

i. Mirena IUS

j. Vaginal hysterectomy

For each scenario described below, choose the SINGLE most likely treatment option from the above list of options. Each option may be used once, more than once, or not at all.

4. A 65-year-old woman has noticed leakage of urine on coughing and sneezing. She has no urgency or frequency. A urine dipstick and culture is negative, but examination reveals a small cystocele. You refer her for urodynamics which shows stress incontinence. Pelvic floor exercises have not helped and she has decided she does not want surgery.

5. A 46-year-old woman gives a history of heavy periods for 3 years. She had previously tried a Mirena IUS but, due to its expulsion, she has been put off the idea of an IUS. An ultrasound scan shows no pathology and a Pipelle endometrial sample is normal. She has 3 children and feels her family is complete. As she has started a new job she is reluctant to take too much time off work.

6. A 51-year-old woman has a history of menorrhagia for the past 6 years. She has a 16 week sized fibroid uterus which is causing her to have urinary frequency and some bowel symptoms.

7–10. What is your diagnosis?

a. Sheehan syndrome

b. Turner syndrome

c. Androgen insensitivity syndrome

d. Congenital adrenal hyperplasia

e. Mayer–Rokitansky–Küster–Hauser syndrome = mullarian agenesis

f. Premature ovarian insufficiency

g. Prolactinoma

h. Polycystic ovarian syndrome

For each scenario described below, choose the SINGLE most likely diagnosis from the above list of options. Each option may be used once, more than once, or not at all.

7. A 15-year-old girl attends with her mother who is concerned as she has not yet started her periods. On examination you notice she is short and does not have

development of breasts, pubic or axillary hair. 'Streak ovaries' are mentioned on an ultrasound scan.

8. A 30-year-old woman attends clinic with a history of menstrual irregularity and difficulty in conceiving. She mentions having headaches and has noticed some leaking from her nipples.

9. A 35-year-old woman attends with secondary amenorrhoea. She had a baby 1 year ago and has not had a period since her delivery. She mentions that she had lost a lot of blood following delivery and struggled to breastfeed her baby afterwards.

10. A 16-year-old attends your clinic and is worried as she has not yet started her periods. On examination, she is of normal height and has normal breast and pubic hair development. On an ultrasound scan, a uterus cannot be seen.

11–15.   What is the most appropriate UKMEC category:

   a.   UKMEC3

   b.   UKMEC4

   c.   UKMEC3 continuation

   d.   UKMEC2 continuation

   e.   UKMEC2 initiation

   f.   UKMEC4 continuation

   g.   UKMEC3 initiation

For each scenario described below, choose the SINGLE most likely UKMEC category from the above list of options. Each option may be used once, more than once, or not at all.

11. A 34-year-old woman with a history of cardiomyopathy with impaired cardiac function requests the combined pill.

12. A 26-year-old woman has recently had a surgical uterine evacuation procedure for a molar pregnancy. Her hCG levels have been found to be decreasing and she requests an IUD for contraception.

13. A 28-year-old woman with active viral hepatitis wishes to continue using the combined patch.

14. A 42-year-old woman is being treated for pelvic tuberculosis. She has an IUS *in situ* which she wishes to continue using.

15. A 23-year-old woman is requesting an emergency IUD. She is found to be chlamydia-positive but does not have any symptoms.

16–17. What is the most likely diagnosis:

    a. Postnatal blues

    b. Anxiety

    c. Puerperal psychosis

    d. Postnatal depression

    e. Bipolar disorder

For each scenario described below, choose the SINGLE most likely diagnosis from the above list of options. Each option may be used once, more than once, or not at all.

16. Amanda is a 32-year-old woman who had a normal delivery 3 weeks ago. She attends with her mother who tells you that within the first few days of delivery Amanda has seemed quite restless, confused and agitated. Amanda tells you she has been hearing voices and has been struggling to sleep.

17. Lucy is a 29-year-old woman who had her first baby 4 days ago. Her mood has been fluctuating and she has been feeling mainly tearful and anxious but has also been irritable over trivial things. She has no other significant history.

18–20. What is the most appropriate term?

    a. Case-based discussion

    b. DOPS (directly observed procedural skill)

    c. Appraisal

    d. OSAT   *objective structured assessment of skills*

    e. Assessment

    f. Mini-CEX (mini clinical evaluation exercise)

For each description below, choose the SINGLE most likely term from the above list of options. Each option may be used once, more than once, or not at all.

18. A structured format which establishes learning goals, addresses concerns in a supportive way and which uses certain objectives against which the progress of the trainee is monitored.

19. A test which measures learning and to see whether competency has been achieved by the trainee.

20. An assessment tool which can be used in both formative and summative encounters.

21–24. What is the most appropriate term?

    a. Pendleton's rules

    b. Reliability

    c. Miller's pyramid

    d. Validity

    e. Maslow's hierarchy of needs

    f. Bloom's taxonomy of educational objectives

For each description below, choose the SINGLE most likely term from the above list of options. Each option may be used once, more than once, or not at all.

21. A model showing gradual progress to eventual attainment or mastering a skill.

22. Determination of the ability of an assessment tool to measure what it was intended to measure.

23. Encompasses three domains – cognitive domain (knowledge), affective domain (attitudes), psychomotor domain (skills).

24. A structure for providing constructive feedback where the trainee also plays an active role.

25–28. What is the correct term?

    a. Caldicott guardian

    b. Implied consent

    c. Clinical effectiveness

    d. Beneficence

    e. Confidentiality

    f. Bolam principle

    g. Clinical supervisor

For each description below, choose the SINGLE most likely term from the above list of options. Each option may be used once, more than once, or not at all.

25. You are the doctor in an outpatient setting and a patient offers you her arm for venepuncture.

26. This is one of the four principles of medical ethics.

27. This is a senior person who is responsible for protecting confidentiality of a patient and service user information and enabling appropriate information sharing.

28. A medical practitioner is not negligent if he or she acts in accordance with a practice that is accepted by a responsible body of medical opinion.

29–31. What is the most appropriate option?

    a. IUD

    b. Pregnancy test in 3 weeks

    c. Double dose levonorgestrel emergency contraception

    d. Ulipristal acetate emergency contraception

    e. Standard dose levonorgestrel emergency contraception

    f. IUS

For each scenario described below, choose the SINGLE most likely term from the above list of options. Each option may be used once, more than once, or not at all.

29. A 25-year-old woman had one episode of unprotected sex 30 hours ago. Her last menstrual period was 10 days ago and her cycles are usually 28 days. She declines an IUD as she dislikes the thought of anything 'in her body', but would like to start an oral contraceptive method today for future contraception. Her BMI is 28.

30. A 32-year-old woman has attended clinic today for emergency contraception. She had unprotected sex 24 hours ago. Her last period was 15 days ago and her cycles are 28 days long. She tells you she is taking carbamazepine and would like ongoing contraception today.

31. A 28-year-old woman had unprotected sex 80 hours ago. Her last period was 13 days ago and her cycles are 30 days long. She says this was a 'fling' with a work colleague which will not happen again. She does not want any ongoing contraceptive method as her husband has had a vasectomy.

32–35. What is the most appropriate management option?

    a. Vaginal hysterectomy

    b. Ring pessary

    c. Antimuscarinic therapy

    d. Anterior colporrhaphy

    e. Posterior colpoperineorrhaphy

    f. Pelvic floor muscle training

    g. Abdominal hysterectomy

For each scenario described below, choose the SINGLE most appropriate management option from the above list of options. Each option may be used once, more than once, or not at all.

32. A 34-year-old woman attends clinic with concerns of leaking urine during exercise. She used to go jogging frequently but, due to the leaking, has stopped doing so. She has 2 children born by vaginal deliveries, and does not want any more. She does not have any significant medical history.

33. A 59-year-old woman had been complaining of a bulge in her vagina. The examination findings mentioned uterocervical descent with the cervix visible at the introitus. She is sexually active and has various medical conditions including chronic obstructive pulmonary disease (COPD).

34. A 60-year-old woman attends your clinic and tells you she can feel a bulge in her vagina. She has also been struggling frequently to pass urine and, whenever she goes to the toilet, she feels as if her bladder is not completely empty. You examine her and document the presence of a cystocele in your notes.

35. A 56-year-old woman tells you she has to pass urine up to 10 times a day and has to wake up once or twice in the night too. Often she feels she needs to get to the toilet quickly otherwise she may have an accident (leakage of urine). She wears pads whenever she is out of the house but tries to avoid going anywhere due to fear of leaking urine.

36–39. What is the most likely diagnosis?

    a. Genital herpes infection

    b. Molluscum contagiosum

    c. Genital warts

    d. Secondary syphilis

    e. Lymphogranuloma venereum

    f. Infected hair follicles

    g. Primary syphilis

    h. HIV

    i. *Trichomonas vaginalis*

For each scenario described below, choose the SINGLE most appropriate diagnosis from the above list of options. Each option may be used once, more than once, or not at all.

36. A 27-year-old woman has noticed 15–20 lumps scattered over her mons pubis area; they are not painful but can be itchy at times. On examination you find smooth, pearly papules of 3mm size with a central umbilication.

37. A 30-year-old woman attends the GUM clinic complaining of vaginal soreness and a frothy yellow discharge for the past week. On a wet smear of the discharge, you see a flagellated organism.

38. A 28-year-old male attends your clinic feeling generally unwell. He tells you that he regularly has sex with other men. He has a rash over his trunk and back and also on his palms and the soles of his feet. When you examine inside his mouth, you notice serpiginous ulcers with a white/grey border.

39. A 29-year-old woman, who arrived in the UK from Zimbabwe 4 months ago, attends clinic feeling generally unwell and complaining of loss of appetite, night sweats and tiredness. When you examine her mouth, you notice white patches on her tongue and over her palate.

40–42. What is the most likely diagnosis?

    a. Primary syphilis

    b. Donovanosis

    c. Lymphogranuloma venereum

    d. Chancroid

    e. Trauma

    f. Genital herpes

    g. Gonorrhoea

For each scenario described below, choose the SINGLE most appropriate diagnosis from the above list of options. Each option may be used once, more than once, or not at all.

40. A 28-year-old man returned from a holiday to Mozambique 10 days ago. He mentions he had vaginal sex with a sex worker there. For the past couple of days he has noticed an ulcer on the glans area of his penis. On examination you see an ulcer with a ragged undermined edge and a greyish base which bleeds easily on touch. Microscopy of a Gram-stained smear of material from the ulcer base shows Gram-negative coccobacilli with occasional chaining.

41. A 32-year-old woman has recently arrived in the UK from Papua New Guinea and attends your clinic saying that she has noticed an area on her labia that was initially a nodule but has now become an ulcer. It isn't painful but she finds the appearance of it distressing. On examination you notice a 'beefy-red' ulcer with rolled edges. A tissue biopsy with Giemsa stain reveals rod-shaped inclusion bodies in the cytoplasm of macrophages.

42. A 26-year-old woman attends clinic complaining of soreness all over her vulva. She tells you she had flu-like symptoms for a week, after which she noticed tingling and discomfort in her genital area and in her legs too. For the past 2 days she has now seen blisters and sores all over her vulva. On examination you notice tender inguinal lymphadenopathy and extensive bilateral crops of blisters and ulcers over the labia majora and minora.

43–45. What is the most appropriate treatment?

    a. Imiquimod

    b. Aciclovir

    c. Podophyllotoxin

    d. Cryotherapy

    e. Ultra-potent topical steroid

    f. Metronidazole

    g. Azithromycin

For each scenario described below, choose the SINGLE most appropriate treatment from the above list of options. Each option may be used once, more than once, or not at all.

43. A 24-year-old woman attends clinic complaining of a smelly vaginal discharge for the past week. You examine her and find a raised vaginal pH of >4.5 and clue cells are noted on microscopy.

44. A 29-year-old woman has noticed lumps in her vulval area for the past 2 weeks. They are numerous and can be itchy at times. You examine her and see multiple soft, flesh-coloured lumps over the labia majora and perianal area. She is 26 weeks pregnant.

45. A 58-year-old woman gives a history of vulval itching and soreness for the past 8 months. It has gradually worsened and she now finds it difficult to have sex with her partner. On examination, you notice pale white atrophic areas on the vulva and also in the perianal area. You cannot see the labia minora and there is midline fusion which makes it difficult to identify the normal architecture.

46–49. What is the most appropriate term?

    a. Commissioning

    b. Health needs assessment

    c. Business case

    d. Quantitative patient survey

    e. Surveillance

    f. Qualitative patient survey

    g. Screening

For each description below, choose the SINGLE most likely term from the above list of options. Each option may be used once, more than once, or not at all.

46. Ensuring the right information is available at the right time and in the right place to inform public health action, programme planning and evaluation and for formulating research hypotheses.

47. The process of identifying healthy people who may be at increased risk of disease or conditions.

48. A systematic method of identifying unmet health and healthcare needs of a population and making changes to meet those unmet needs.

49. This term encompasses many actions ranging from health needs assessment for a population, to service specification and contract negotiation or procurement, with continuous quality assessment.

50–52. Select the term which best describes each of these scenarios:

    a. Consensual sex

    b. Rape

    c. Sexual activity with a child

    d. Sexual assault

    e. Assault by penetration

    f. Drug-facilitated sexual assault

50. A 28-year-old woman mentions that her 45-year-old male boss had tried to kiss her and touch her breasts after a meeting in his office. This happened in spite of her telling him to stop.

51. A 16-year-old female has recently started a relationship with an 18-year-old male. They had oral and vaginal intercourse which she agreed to.

52. A 25-year-old woman had been to a party where she had a lot to drink. She has only partial memory of events from earlier in the evening when she was chatting to a 30-year-old man but cannot remember events after that. She is shocked to have woken up in his bed and he says he had vaginal intercourse with her.

53–55. Select the most appropriate term for each of the following scenarios:

    a. Placenta percreta

    b. Placenta increta

    c. Retained products of conception

    d. Placenta praevia

    e. Vasa praevia

    f. Sepsis

    g. Placental abruption

53. A woman attends antenatal clinic and is 32 weeks pregnant. Her routine anomaly scan at 20 weeks of gestation had shown a low lying placenta covering the internal os. A repeat scan she has had today has shown the same findings. This is her second pregnancy. She has had 1 previous caesarean delivery.

54. A 26-year-old woman had a medical abortion 4 weeks ago. She has been having bleeding most days since the procedure and this is worrying her. She gets occasional lower abdominal cramps but is otherwise well. On transvaginal ultrasound scan you see mixed echogenic material in the endometrial cavity which you measure as being 25mm.

55. A 19-year-old woman had a surgical abortion 5 days ago. She has been admitted feeling unwell and shivery. She mentions having a foul-smelling discharge and on examination is found to have a temperature of >38°C, is tachycardic and has tenderness in her lower abdomen.

56–58. Select the most appropriate contraceptive method choice for each scenario:

a. IUS – 13.5mg

b. IUD

c. Combined pills

d. IUS – 52mg

e. Laparoscopic sterilisation

f. Implant

g. Progestogen-only pill

56. A 34-year-old woman has ulcerative colitis and had undergone an ileal pouch anal anastomosis (IPAA) surgery 6 weeks ago. She has 2 children, both born by caesarean section, and feels her family is complete. She would like effective contraception but is put off by the thought of intrauterine methods.

57. A 28-year-old woman who has SLE attends the community contraceptive clinic requesting contraception. She has no antiphospholipid antibodies and would like to start a contraceptive method today. Her BMI is 35 and she is normotensive. She stopped smoking 8 months ago. Her periods are regular and she tells you she would prefer a regular cycle.

58. A 26-year-old nulliparous woman attends clinic requesting an intrauterine method of contraception. Whilst taking a history, she mentions she had had unexplained episodes of fainting and was referred to the cardiologists. She has been diagnosed with long QT syndrome. She is unable to give you much detail today. She has a history of heavy periods and tells you she wants to start contraception today.

59–62. Select the most appropriate treatment option for each scenario:

a. Sequential HRT (oral preparation)

b. Vagifem 10mcg pessaries

c. Sequential HRT (transdermal preparation)

d. Continuous combined HRT (transdermal preparation)

e. Meditation

f. Continuous combined HRT (oral preparation)

    g. Sandrena gel

    h. Mirtazapine

59. A 63-year-old woman attends your clinic complaining of superficial dyspareunia for the past year which has gradually worsened. She has been avoiding sex for the same reason and this is now affecting her relationship with her partner.

60. A 54-year-old woman has been on HRT for the past 5 years. She has been using an oral preparation with a regular withdrawal bleed. She attends for review. Her BP is normal. Her BMI is 36.

61. A 51-year-old woman has been having hot flushes. She had breast cancer 2 years ago and is on tamoxifen. She tells you that she has cut down on coffee and is exercising more. She wants to know if you can suggest any other treatment option which might improve her symptoms.

62. A 49-year-old woman had a Mirena fitted 1 year ago. She has been getting hot flushes, night sweats which disturb her sleep, and is feeling generally tired and irritable. She would like you to suggest a treatment option to start as soon as possible. She is normotensive and has a BMI of 35. She has no significant medical or family history.

63–66. Select the most appropriate term for each scenario:

    a. Secondary anorgasmia

    b. Retarded ejaculation

    c. Unprovoked vulvodynia

    d. Non consummation

    e. Primary anorgasmia

    f. Psychogenic erectile dysfunction

    g. Provoked vulvodynia

    h. Premature ejaculation

63. A 24-year-old man attends your clinic. He is anxious because he is unable to produce an erection. He has been in a relationship with his current partner for 2 months. He states that this has never happened with previous partners and that he gets early morning erections and is able to maintain an erection during masturbation.

64. A 25-year-old man is being treated for a condition using cognitive behavioural therapy – namely the 'stop–start' technique, and has been using condoms with local anaesthetic. He feels this has helped him but a tablet called dapoxetine which you gave him for this condition has been making him feel nauseous and sleepy.

65. A 29-year-old woman has been with her partner for the past 8 years. She tells you that for the past year she has stopped feeling any sexual excitement during intercourse and is worried about this. She says this all started following an abortion she had 1 year ago. Prior to that she found sex with her partner to be pleasurable and was able to climax. She still struggles with feelings of guilt regarding the abortion and wonders if everything is related.

66. A 30-year-old woman attends clinic feeling very anxious. She has been struggling with a burning and at times sore sensation in her vulval area. It is specifically at the opening of her vagina and is triggered by touch. She has been seen by gynaecologists who have found no reason for her symptoms. This is affecting her relationship and causing her to feel very worried.

67–70. Which is the most appropriate option for the following scenarios?

   a. Oxytocin

   b. Laparoscopic salpingectomy

   c. Beta hCG

   d. Mifepristone

   e. Prostaglandin E2 analogue

   f. Manual vacuum aspiration

   g. Prostaglandin E1 analogue

   h. Methotrexate

67. A 28-year-old woman has a positive urine pregnancy test but does not want to keep the pregnancy. Her last menstrual period was 7 weeks ago and she tells you her periods are usually quite regular. On transvaginal ultrasound scan you see an empty uterus and no obvious pathology.

68. A 19-year-old woman is pregnant but does not want to keep the pregnancy. She attends your morning clinic requesting an abortion method which will allow her to have it 'all sorted today'. She is at 8 weeks of gestation on transvaginal scan.

69. A 26-year-old woman gives a history of a positive urine pregnancy test and says she has had some light vaginal bleeding for the past 2 days. The beta hCG result is 6000 and on transvaginal ultrasound scan you see an empty uterus and some free fluid in the pouch of Douglas. There is right adnexal mass (38mm in size) with a foetal heart present.

70. A 33-year-old woman is having a medical abortion at 7 weeks of gestation and has attended for her second visit today. At her first visit she had been given an oral tablet to commence the abortion process. Today you give her a medication which, apart from abortion, has been used in the prevention of NSAID-induced gastric ulcers and management of postpartum bleeding.

71–74. Select the most appropriate option from the list below for each scenario:

a. Clinical audit

b. The Ombudsman

c. Clinical effectiveness

d. Incident reporting

e. Research

f. Root cause analysis

g. CPD

h. Judicial review

71. This is a procedure that allows a court of law to review decisions made by public bodies. Patients can make a claim for this if they feel they have been directly affected by an unlawful act or decision of an NHS body.

72. The process of identifying what went wrong after an event has occurred. It involves an investigation team gathering data and putting together a chronology of events to identify care delivery problems and contributory factors.

73. A quality improvement process which seeks to improve patient care and outcomes through systematic review of care against explicit criteria and the implementation of change.

74. A continuing process, outside formal undergraduate and postgraduate training, that enables individual doctors to maintain and improve standards of medical practice through the development of knowledge, skills, attitudes and behaviour.

75–77. Select the most appropriate term for each scenario:

    a. Urinary hormone monitoring

    b. Standard days method

    c. Symptothermal method

    d. Cervical secretions monitoring

    e. Lactational amenorrhoea

    f. Two day method

    g. Calendar method

75. A 32-year-old woman is keen to try a particular fertility awareness method for contraception which combines various fertility indicators. You explain to her that with perfect use of this method, pregnancy rates at 1 year are 0.4%.

76. A 28-year-old woman delivered a baby 8 weeks ago. She is exclusively breastfeeding and has not yet had a period. She states she is relying on this for contraception.

77. A 26-year-old woman has epilepsy which is well controlled on sodium valproate. She has heard from a friend that a fertility monitoring device called Persona is available which can be used for contraception and she has come to discuss this. You explain to her that this particular method would not be suitable due to the medication that she is on and its potential teratogenic effects.

78–80. Select the most appropriate diagnosis for each scenario:

    a. Ovarian torsion

    b. Ovarian hyperstimulation syndrome

    c. Ectopic pregnancy

    d. Pelvic inflammatory disease

    e. Endometriosis

    f. Sepsis

78. A 27-year-old woman attends A&E with abdominal pain, nausea and vomiting. She has been undergoing IVF treatment but a urine pregnancy test is negative. On ultrasound scan, there is evidence of ascites and the ovaries are enlarged to 9cm in size.

79. A 24-year-old woman attends feeling unwell and feverish. She complains of deep dyspareunia and a foul-smelling discharge for the past few days. On examination, she is found to be pyrexial and tachycardic, with lower abdominal tenderness. On speculum examination you notice a mucopurulent cervicitis and when you examine her bimanually, there is cervical excitation.

80. A 29-year-old woman attends with severe lower abdominal pain of sudden onset. She does not have any troublesome vaginal discharge but tells you she has a dermoid cyst on her left ovary and is awaiting surgery on this. She looks unwell and on examination she is found to have a raised temperature, is hypotensive and tachycardic.

Answers to EMQs

Answers to questions 1–3

Suggested reading:

Michala and Creighton. Fused labia: a paediatric approach. *TOG*, 2009;11:261.

Paediatric and Adolescent Gynaecology for the MRCOG and Beyond – www.britspag.org

RCOG online learning modules – https://stratog.rcog.org.uk

1. Correct response   **C**   Imperforate hymen

2. Correct response   **A**   Labial adhesions

3. Correct response   **B**   Bartholin's cyst

Answers to questions 4–6

Suggested reading:

NICE, *Heavy menstrual bleeding*. CG44, 2007.

NICE, *Urinary incontinence in women*. CG171, 2016.

4. Correct response   **B**   Duloxetine

5. Correct response   **H**   Endometrial ablation

6. Correct response   **D**   Total abdominal hysterectomy

Answers to questions 7–10

Suggested reading:

UpToDate, *Evaluation and management of primary amenorrhea*. October 2016.

UpToDate, *Evaluation and management of secondary amenorrhea*. August 2016.

7. Correct response   **B**   Turner syndrome

8. Correct response   **G**   Prolactinoma

9. Correct response   **A**   Sheehan syndrome

10. Correct response   **E**   Mayer–Rokitansky–Küster–Hauser syndrome

Answers to questions 11–15

Suggested reading:

FSRH, *Contraception after pregnancy*. January 2017.

FSRH, *Contraceptive choices for women with cardiac disease*. June 2014.

FSRH, *Intrauterine contraception*. April 2015.

UKMEC, 2016.

11. Correct response   **B**   UKMEC4

12. Correct response   **A**   UKMEC3

13. Correct response   **D**   UKMEC2 continuation

14. Correct response   **F**   UKMEC4 continuation

15. Correct response   **G**   UKMEC3 initiation

Answers to questions 16–17

Suggested reading:

NICE, *Routine postnatal care of women and their babies*. CG37, 2015.

16. Correct response   **C**   Puerperal psychosis

17. Correct response   **A**   Postnatal blues

Answers to questions 18–20

Suggested reading:

General Medical Council, *Leadership and Management for All Doctors*. GMC, 2012.

Parry-Smith, Mahmud, Landau and Hayes, Workplace-based assessment: a new approach to existing tools. *TOG*, 2014;16:281.

RCOG online learning modules – https://stratog.rcog.org.uk

18. Correct response   **C**   Appraisal

19. Correct response   **E**   Assessment

20. Correct response   **D**   OSAT

Answers to questions 21–24

Suggested reading:

Duthie and Garden, The teacher, the learner and the method. *TOG*, 2010;12:273.

www.gp-training.net/training/educational_theory/index.htm

21. Correct response   **C**   Miller's pyramid

22. Correct response   **D**   Validity

23. Correct response   **F**   Bloom's taxonomy of educational objectives

24. Correct response   **A**   Pendleton's rules

Answers to questions 25–28

Suggested reading:

RCOG, *Obtaining valid consent*. CGA6, 2015.

GMC, *Good medical practice*. 2013.

25. Correct response   **B**   Implied consent

26. Correct response   **D**   Beneficence

27. Correct response   **A**   Caldicott guardian

28. Correct response   **F**   Bolam principle

Answers to questions 29–31

Suggested reading:

FSRH, *Clinical guidance: emergency contraception*. March 2017.

29. Correct response   **C**   Double dose levonorgestrel emergency contraception

30. Correct response   **A**   IUD

31. Correct response   **D**   Ulipristal acetate emergency contraception

Answers to questions 32–35

Suggested reading:

NICE, *Urinary incontinence in women: management.* CG171, 2016.

32. Correct response   **F**   Pelvic floor muscle training

33. Correct response   **B**   Ring pessary

34. Correct response   **D**   Anterior colporrhaphy

35. Correct response   **C**   Antimuscarinic therapy

Answers to questions 36–39

Suggested reading:

BASHH, *Molluscum contagiosum.* 2014.

BASHH, *Trichomonas vaginalis.* 2014.

BASHH, *Syphilis.* 2015.

RCGP, *Sexually transmitted infections in primary care.* 2013.

36. Correct response   **B**   Molluscum contagiosum

37. Correct response   **I**   *Trichomonas vaginalis*

38. Correct response   **D**   Secondary syphilis

39. Correct response   **H**   HIV

Answers to questions 40–42

Suggested reading:

BASHH, *Genital ulceration.* 2014.

40. Correct response   **D**   Chancroid

41. Correct response   **B**   Donovanosis

42. Correct response   **F**   Genital herpes

Answers to questions 43–45

Suggested reading:

RCGP, *Sexually transmitted infections in primary care*. 2013.

RCOG, *Management of vulval skin disorders*. GTG58, 2011.

43. Correct response   **F**   Metronidazole

44. Correct response   **D**   Cryotherapy

45. Correct response   **E**   Ultra-potent topical steroid

Answers to questions 46–49

Suggested reading:

DoH, *Public health surveillance: towards a public health surveillance strategy for England*. 2012.

www.england.nhs.uk/commissioning

www.healthknowledge.org.uk/public-health-textbook

46. Correct response   **E**   Surveillance

47. Correct response   **G**   Screening

48. Correct response   **B**   Health needs assessment

49. Correct response   **A**   Commissioning

Answers to questions 50–52

Suggested reading:

The Sexual Offences Act: www.legislation.gov.uk/ukpga/2003/42/contents

50. Correct response   **D**   Sexual assault

51. Correct response   **A**   Consensual sex

52. Correct response   **B**   Rape

Answers to questions 53–55

Suggested reading:

RCOG, *Best practice in comprehensive abortion care*. BPP2, 2015.

RCOG, *Placenta praevia, placenta praevia accreta and vasa praevia: diagnosis and management*. GTG27, 2011.

RCOG, *The care of women requesting induced abortion*. EBCG7, 2011.

53. Correct response   **D**   Placenta praevia

54. Correct response   **C**   Retained products of conception

55. Correct response   **F**   Sepsis

Answers to questions 56–58

Suggested reading:

FSRH, *CEU Guidance: Contraceptive choices for women with cardiac disease*. June 2014.

FSRH, *CEU Guidance: Sexual and reproductive health for individuals with inflammatory bowel disease*. October 2016.

UKMEC, 2016.

56. Correct response   **F**   Implant

57. Correct response   **B**   IUD

58. Correct response   **G**   Progestogen-only pill

Answers to questions 59–62

Suggested reading:

NICE, *Menopause: diagnosis and management*, CG23, Nov 2015

59. Correct response   **B**   Vagifem 10mcg pessaries

60. Correct response   **D**   Continuous combined HRT (transdermal preparation)

61. Correct response   **H**   Mirtazapine

62. Correct response   **G**   Sandrena gel

Answers to questions 63–66

Suggested reading:

Cowan and Frodsham, Common disorders in psychosexual medicine. *TOG*, 2015;17:47.

63. Correct response	**F**	Psychogenic erectile dysfunction
64. Correct response	**H**	Premature ejaculation
65. Correct response	**A**	Secondary anorgasmia
66. Correct response	**G**	Provoked vulvodynia

Answers to questions 67–70

Suggested reading:

NICE, *Ectopic pregnancy and miscarrriage: diagnosis and initial management in early pregnancy of ectopic pregnancy and miscarriage.* CG154, 2012.

RCOG, *Diagnosis and management of ectopic pregnancy.* GTG21, 2016.

RCOG, *The care of women requesting induced abortion.* EBCG7, 2011.

67. Correct response	**C**	Beta hCG
68. Correct response	**F**	Manual vacuum aspiration
69. Correct response	**B**	Laparascopic salpingectomy
70. Correct response	**G**	Prostaglandin E1 analogue

Answers to questions 71–74

Suggested reading:

RCOG, *Improving patient safety: risk management for maternity and gynaecology.* CGA No. 2, 2009.

RCOG, *Understanding audit.* CGA No. 5, 2003.

71. Correct response	**H**	Judicial review
72. Correct response	**F**	Root cause analysis
73. Correct response	**A**	Clinical audit
74. Correct response	**G**	CPD

Answers to questions 75–77

Suggested reading:

FSRH, *CEU Guidance: Fertility awareness methods.* June 2015 (updated November 2015).

75. Correct response   **C**   Symptothermal method

76. Correct response   **E**   Lactational amenorrhoea

77. Correct response   **A**   Urinary hormone monitoring

Answers to questions 78–80

Suggested reading:

BASHH, *UK National Guideline for the Management of Pelvic Inflammatory Disease.* 2011.

RCOG, *The management of ovarian hyperstimulation syndrome.* GTG5, Feb 2016.

RCOG online learning modules – https://stratog.rcog.org.uk

78. Correct response   **B**   Ovarian hyperstimulation syndrome

79. Correct response   **D**   Pelvic inflammatory disease

80. Correct response   **A**   Ovarian torsion

Hints and tips for the Critical Reading Questions paper

The CRQ section of the exam often causes considerable anxiety. The aim of this part of the exam is to ensure that candidates are equipped with the skills necessary to read a scientific paper, appraise the research and determine whether the results will inform their clinical practice. Evidence hierarchy reflects the authority of different types of research. Randomised controlled trials are the gold standard, with systematic reviews, meta-analyses and observational studies being ranked as less influential. This hierarchy of evidence forms the basis for evidence-based medicine.

The CRQ is a 90 minute written paper which is divided into three sections.

All or parts of an academic paper may be given to you and you will be expected to answer five to ten questions on each part. You may also be given a statistical diagram, such as a forest plot, a box and whisker diagram, scatter diagram, etc. that you will be required to interpret and answer questions on.

The CRQ forms 33.3% of the marks of the whole examination.

The most common question that candidates ask in relation to the CRQ paper is "How do I revise for it?". It is important to be aware of different types of study design and methodology and how this influences the clinical impact of a study. You need to read as many clinical papers from different journals as you can and attend a journal club or, if there isn't one already, start your own!

When assessing clinical papers, it is important to use a logical method to appraise the information being presented. To appraise a study, it is helpful to follow the simple PICO mnemonic:

Population

Intervention

Comparison

Outcomes.

The following questions may also be helpful:

1. What is the purpose of the study?

2. What is the research question?

3. What is the study design?

4. What type of statistical analysis has been used?

5. What are the results of the study?

Once you have made the decision to do the membership examination, it is good practice to apply the above questions to all articles that you read. It is good forward planning to commit to critically appraising one clinical paper a week.

A critical appraisal course may be useful, but is not essential to pass this component of the exam. There are various books on critical appraisal, which might be useful – ensure that you have looked at the examples provided on the FSRH website, or consider:

Clinical Evidence Made Easy, Harris, Taylor and Jackson, Scion Publishing.

Medical Statistics Made Easy 3e, Harris and Taylor, Scion Publishing.

Critical Reading Questions - One

This set of questions relate to the following paper:

Effects of injectable progestogen contraception versus the copper intrauterine device on HIV acquisition: sub-study of a pragmatic randomised controlled trial
Hofmeyr, Singata-Madliki, Lawrie, Bergel, Temmerman
J Fam Plann Reprod Health Care, 2017;**43**:175.

Please download a free copy (http://srh.bmj.com/content/43/3/175) and read through before attempting to answer the questions below.

1. What is the research question?

2. Describe the study undertaken.
   - What was the experimental intervention?

3. What is the primary outcome?

4. Are any secondary outcomes considered?

5. List the limitations of this observational study.

6. List and discuss the statistical tests applied to the data in this study.

Critical Reading Questions - Two

This set of questions relate to the following paper:

Practice and intention to use long acting and permanent contraceptive methods among married women in Ethiopia: systematic meta-analysis
Mesfin and Kibret
Reproductive Health 2016;13:78.

Please download a free copy (https://reproductive-health-journal.biomedcentral. com/articles/10.1186/s12978-016-0194-0/open-peer-review) and read through before attempting to answer the questions below.

1. What is a systematic meta-analysis? Relate your answer to the clinical paper provided.

2. What were the exclusion criteria for this study?

   Helpful tip:
   The pooled estimated prevalence rates for intention to use and actual use of long acting or permanent contraception are provided with 95% confidence intervals. This means that the selected samples have a 0.95 probability of reflecting the population mean (95% chance of reflecting the population mean).

3. Look at *Figure 2* in the paper and answer the following questions:
   a. What is the name of this type of diagram?
   b. What is the significance of the large diamond? What do its horizontal points tell you?
   c. What do the small black squares represent?
   d. What is the significance of the small horizontal black lines associated with each black square?
   e. What is the significance of the dark vertical line?
   f. Is the combined result of this meta-analysis statistically significant? How can you tell this from the diagram?
   g. Looking at *Figure 2*, what was the pooled prevalence of intention to use long acting permanent contraceptive methods among married women?
   h. What does 95% confidence interval mean?
   i. Which study in *Figure 2* has the smallest confidence interval?

4. What were the limitations of this study?

5. What analysis was used to assess heterogeneity?

Critical Reading Questions - Three

This set of questions relate to the following figure:

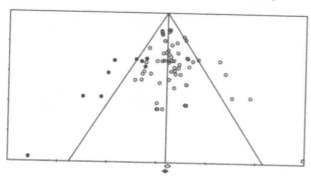

1. What type of diagram is shown?

2. Why might this type of diagram be used?

3. What does each dot in this diagram represent?

4. What is the significance of the shape of this diagram?

5. What is meant by the term "publication bias"?

6. What test can be done to check for asymmetry?

7. What do the *x* and *y* axes show?

Critical Reading Questions - Four

This set of questions relate to the following figure:

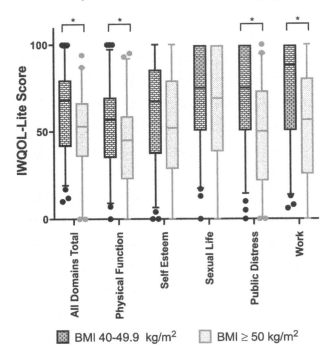

Image reproduced from:
Weight-related quality of life in obese, pregnant women in South Africa
Tisane, Van der Merwe and Hal. *J Endocrinol, Metab Diabetes South Africa* 2017;22:43.

1. What type of diagram is shown?

2. What does the horizontal line in each box represent?

3. What is the significance of the top and bottom of each box?

4. What does each box represent?

5. What is the significance of the vertical lines coming from each box?

6. What is the significance of the dots above and below the vertical lines seen in this diagram?

Critical Reading Questions - Five

This set of questions relate to the following figure:

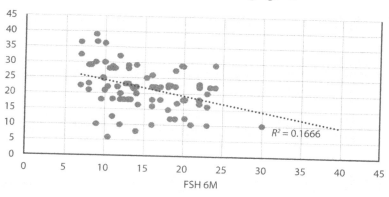

FSH 6M

Image reproduced from:

Study on the change in function of the preserved ovaries following hysterectomy by abdominal versus vaginal route

Dasgupta, Jha, Naskar, Bag and Biswas. *Andrology and Gynecology: Current Research*, 2017;5:1 (*doi: 10.4172/2327-4360.1000157*).

This diagram represents ovarian blood flow in preserved ovaries following hysterectomy, by either a vaginal or abdominal route, 6 months after the procedure (V_{max} 6M vertical axis). The horizontal axis reflects the impact of surgery on preserved ovarian function – reflected by follicle stimulating hormone (FSH 6M) level – increases with loss of ovarian function.

1. What is the name of this diagram?

2. What is the significance of this type of diagram?

3. Describe the overall result displayed on the diagram.

4. What is the significance of R^2? What is it also known as?

Answers to CRQs

Answers to CRQ One

1. What is the research question?
Does use of DMPA increase HIV acquisition rates?

2. Describe the study undertaken.
Pragmatic, open label, parallel-arm, randomised controlled trial (RCT) comparing IUC and injectable progestogen in relation to pregnancy rates and HIV acquisition rates.
- What was the experimental intervention?

Voluntary HIV testing offered at baseline, coinciding with delivery of either a Cu-IUD or an injectable progestin and with further HIV testing 12 or more months later.

3. What is the primary outcome?
Primary outcome: pregnancy.

4. Are any secondary outcomes considered?
Secondary outcome: HIV acquisition.

5. List the limitations of this observational study.
Sample size – too small to have adequate power to detect the hypothesised effect (that HIV acquisition rates are higher in women using injectable progestins for contraception). $P = 0.7$ – suggests that the findings could be due to chance.

Additional notes:
Null hypothesis – *any difference in the groups being compared is due to chance.*
Confidence intervals – *the confidence interval gives the range in which the true value is likely to be found.*
***P* value** *(statistical significance) – the* P *value for significance is most commonly set at 0.05.* P *values tell us the probability that chance was the reason for the results. A smaller* P *value indicates a lesser likelihood of the results having been achieved by chance.*

6. List and discuss the statistical tests applied to the data in this study.
A chi-squared test – used to test the significance of independent categorical data. It tests the null hypothesis that the distribution of a discontinuous variable is the same in the independent groups, in this case that the rate of HIV acquisition is the same with the Cu-IUD and injectable progestin.

A Fisher's exact test – used to test the significance of independent categorical data. It is used as an alternative to the chi-squared test when the sample size is small.

Answers to CRQ Two

1. What is a systematic meta-analysis? Relate your answer to the clinical paper provided.

    A **systematic** review of **cross-sectional** studies (specific subset of the population – in this case women intending to use or using long acting or permanent contraception). The researchers started with 328 articles. Only 16 of these articles were found to be suitable for the final meta-analysis.

    Meta-analysis – statistical synthesis of the results of several (in this case 16) clinical trials all considering the same question (in this case the intention to use and actual use of long acting or permanent methods of contraception).

2. What were the exclusion criteria for this study?
    Studies were excluded from this meta-analysis if:

    a. Articles were focused on short term contraceptives, existing meta-analysis or systematic reviews.

    b. Articles consisted of comments, editorials or duplicate publication of the same study.

    c. Response rate was less than 80%, articles available only in abstract form and articles with sample size of less than 50.

3. Look at *Figure 2* in the paper and answer the following questions:

    a. What is the name of this type of diagram?

    This is a Forest plot, otherwise known as a 'Blobbogram'.

    b. What is the significance of the large diamond? What do its horizontal points tell you?

    The large diamond represents the overall outcome of the meta-analysis and shows the point estimate and confidence intervals when you combine all the individual studies together.

    The horizontal points of the diamond represent the 95% confidence interval of this combined point estimate.

    c. What do the small black squares represent?

    The small black squares represent the point estimate of the study result. The size of the box provides an indication of the size of the study and the weight given to each study in the meta-analysis.

    d. What is the significance of the small horizontal black lines associated with each black square?

The horizontal line represents the 95% confidence intervals of the study result with each end of the line representing the boundaries of the confidence interval.

e. What is the significance of the dark vertical line?

The bold vertical line represents the line of no effect. This line is placed where there is no association between an exposure and an outcome or no difference between 2 interventions.

f. Is the combined result of this meta-analysis statistically significant? How can you tell this from the diagram?

The combined result is statistically significant as the horizontal tips of the diamond do not cross the line of no effect.

g. Looking at *Figure 2*, what was the pooled prevalence of intention to use long acting permanent contraceptive methods among married women?

The pooled prevalence of intention to use LAPCMs among married women was 42.98%.

h. What does 95% confidence interval mean?

The 95% confidence interval is a range of values that you can be 95% certain contain the true mean of the population.

i. Which study in *Figure 2* has the smallest confidence interval?

In *Figure 2*, the Ethiopian DHS 2011 study has the narrowest confidence interval.

4. What were the limitations of this study?
The main limitation is with regard to the representation of the population. The analysis was based on limited studies which were conducted in women who had different socio-cultural and economic characteristics. This might have affected their intention to use and use of LAPCMs.

5. What analysis was used to assess heterogeneity?
Heterogeneity across all studies included in the meta-analysis was estimated using Cochran's Q-test and I^2 test.

Answers to CRQ Three

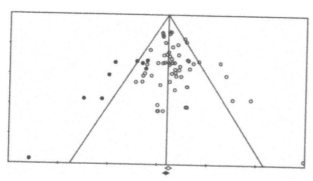

1. What type of diagram is shown here?
   Funnel plot.

2. Why might this type of diagram be used?
   Funnel plots can be used to check whether publication bias exists and they are commonly used in systematic reviews and meta-analyses.

3. What does each dot in this diagram represent?
   A single study.

4. What is the significance of the shape of this diagram?
   The scatter of the dots seen here reflects a symmetrical inverted funnel shape. This indicates an absence of publication bias. It can be assumed that high precision studies will be plotted near the average and low precision studies will show an even spread on both sides of the average. This creates the typical funnel shape.

5. What is meant by the term "publication bias"?
   Research studies showing positive findings have a higher chance of publication when compared with those showing negative findings. This would obviously distort and bias any results from meta-analyses and literature reviews which rely only on published data. This can be compensated for by the inclusion of evidence from unpublished studies in any meta-analysis.

6. What test can be done to check for asymmetry?
   Egger test.

7. What do the x and y axes show?
   x axis – study result.
   y axis – study precision.

Answers to CRQ Four

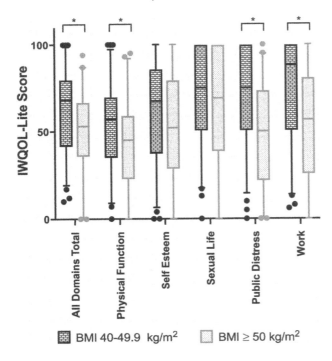

1. What type of diagram is shown?
   Box and whisker plot.

2. What does the horizontal line in each box represent?
   The median value.

3. What is the significance of the top and bottom of each box?
   These represent the upper and lower quartiles of the population being studied (75% and 25%, respectively).

4. What does each box represent?
   The interquartile range.

5. What is the significance of the vertical lines coming from each box?
   These represent the maximum and minimum values, excluding any outliers.

6. What is the significance of the dots above and below the vertical lines seen in this diagram?
   The dots after the end point of each whisker represent any extreme values or outliers.

Answers to CRQ Five

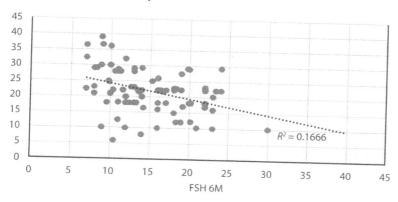

1. What is the name of this diagram?
   The diagram is a scatter plot.

2. What is the significance of this type of diagram?
   A scatter plot helps one determine if a linear relationship exists between two variables – in this case hysterectomy (by whatever route) and the impact of surgery on ovarian function.

3. Describe the overall result displayed on the diagram.
   There is a decrease in ovarian blood flow (V_{max}) "trend", compared with an increase in FSH levels, 6 months after hysterectomy with conservation of the ovaries. This represents a negative correlation, reflecting deterioration in function of conserved ovaries at the time of hysterectomy.

4. What is the significance of R^2? What is it also known as?
   R^2 looks at the spread of the data points around the regression line. It is also called the <u>coefficient</u> of determination.

Hints and tips for the Objective Structured Clinical Examinations

The objective structured clinical examination (OSCE) comprises a circuit of 10 active stations, each lasting 12 minutes. This includes 3 minutes at the start to read the scenario. There may be an additional preparatory station to give the candidate time to get ready for the next station. If more than 10 candidates are in a circuit, there may be a 'rest' station.

The OSCE stations present you with simulations of 'real life' consultations and you will be tested on your performance in various domains. These include data gathering, communication skills, demonstration of person-centred care and your ability to apply your theoretical knowledge and make evidence-based decisions.

Notebooks and pens will be given to you prior to starting the circuit.

The marking is objective and the examiners will have a marking sheet or a checklist to assess your performance.

- A "study buddy" is useful for practising OSCEs – you can provide one another with feedback and learn from each other.
- Make the most of the initial 3 minutes of reading time: read the question thoroughly. It may be helpful to write down key points that you want to cover in your history taking.
- Time management is key, so practise (with your study buddy) timing yourselves.
- Don't have fixed ideas about the OSCE station – there may be hidden agendas!
- Try to be systematic in your approach: broadly divide your consultation into three parts:

   Data gathering
   o Be systematic in your approach.
   o Remember the basics – ICE (ideas, concerns, expectations) and the importance of the 'golden minute'. This is when you first meet the patient and it is an opportunity to allow them to speak!
   o Look for verbal and non-verbal cues – acknowledging these may help reveal the agenda of the station.
   o Summarising – helps you to gather your thoughts and allows you to check if you are missing anything.
   o Keep in mind 'red flags' and explore these, e.g. safeguarding issues, post-menopausal bleeding, etc.

Clinical examination
o   A focused and relevant examination is key. Offer a chaperone where needed.

Clinical management
o   You should have an individualised, patient-centred approach in your clinical management plan.
o   Avoid medical jargon.
o   Offer options, e.g. conservative, medical and surgical options, where appropriate.
o   Check that the patient understands the information provided.
o   Discuss follow-up if appropriate.
o   Summarise and offer information, e.g. leaflets and websites.
- Once you have finished your OSCE station, clear your mind and focus on the next station!
- Last but not least – remember these stations reflect what you do on a daily basis. You have worked hard and have the theoretical knowledge. It's time to show the examiners what you have learnt!

OSCE Scenario One

INFORMATION FOR THE DOCTOR:

Christine is a 19-year-old student who attends a community sexual health clinic with her mother. She reports a sexual assault 48 hours ago, by a man unknown to her.

INFORMATION FOR THE PATIENT:

You are Christine and you are a 19-year-old student. You have attended clinic today with your mother because you were sexually assaulted 48 hours ago. The perpetrator was unknown to you.

Your ideas: you still can't believe this has happened to you and you have come to see the doctor in clinic for advice about what to do next.

Your concerns: you don't want to involve the police at this stage. You are worried that you may have caught some serious infections from the perpetrator.

Your expectations: you expect to be given advice from the doctor and for them to address your concerns about infections.

Information to reveal if asked:

You had a regular male partner for 2 years, but split up 6 months ago. You have had no other sexual partners. Your most recent STI screen was 1 year ago.

You attended a friend's birthday party at her apartment and were walking back home when you were sexually assaulted in a side street by an unknown man of African origin. He penetrated you vaginally with his penis, without a condom, and you think he ejaculated. There was no oral or anal contact. You have some superficial scratches and some bruising to your body, but no other injuries.

You had a shower after the assault when you got home. However, your mum did keep the clothes you had been wearing in case they were required for evidence.

You don't want to involve the police at this stage because you don't feel you could handle it emotionally and your priority is making sure the person who raped you hasn't given you any infections.

You drink alcohol occasionally although you hadn't drunk any at this party. You are a non-smoker, have never used drugs and have no significant medical or surgical history. You have never been pregnant and have been on the combined pill for 2 years, with good compliance. You resumed your pill taking 4 days ago after the pill-free week and have not missed any pills. You are not on any medication and have no allergies.

Your mum has been supporting you, but you can see that she is affected by what has happened too. You don't want to burden her with what has happened to you.

TAKING A FOCUSED HISTORY:

Introduce yourself, confirm details, discuss confidentiality and its limits.

Ask if she would like her mother to be present for the consultation.

Tip 1
This is an OSCE where your ability to have a sensitive discussion, showing empathy, will be assessed.

Tip 2
In the station there may be props for you to use such as boxes of tissues, leaflets, etc. so ensure you use these.

Establish ICE – Ideas, Concerns, Expectations
- Why has she come to see you today?
- What is worrying her?
- What are her expectations from this consultation?

History:
Presenting issue: acknowledge any non-verbal cues and respond accordingly.
- **What** happened?
  - o Consensual?
  - o Vaginal, anal, oral contact? Penetration?
  - o Condom used?
  - o Ejaculation?
  - o Injuries?
  - o Capacity to consent? (drugs, alcohol, head injury or learning difficulty?)
- **Who** was the perpetrator?
  - o Known/unknown
  - o Single assailant?
  - o Ethnicity?
  - o HIV status known or unknown?
  - o IV drug user?
- **When** did it happen?
- **Where** did it happen?
- Police informed or not? Does she wish them to be involved?
  - o Showered since incident?
  - o Clothes washed since incident?
  - o Bowels opened? (relevant in cases of anal assault)
  - o How is she coping? Does she have support?

- **Sexual history**: does she have a partner? Regular/casual?
  - o Length of relationship?
  - o When was her most recent STI screen including HIV testing?
  - o Condom usage?
- **Menstrual history**: last menstrual period; cycles
- **Contraception**: which method is she currently using? Pregnancy risk?
- **Obstetric history**: parity; pregnancies? (in this country? usually screened for HIV antenatally in UK)
- **Medical history**: VTE, migraine, liver disease
- **Medication**: enzyme inducing drugs; prescribed/over the counter/herbal remedies.
- **Social history**: smoking, alcohol, recreational drugs, other drugs (e.g. 'smart' drugs used by students)

Offer: height, weight, blood pressure
- Referral to Sexual Assault Referral Centre (SARC).

Discussion:

This will be a busy OSCE because there are lots of points to discuss. Try to keep to time.

Offer to send to **SARC** because they can provide not only a forensic medical examination and follow-up with services such as GUM, but can also support her with access to counselling services if needed.

Explain that even if she does not want to involve the police at present, she can still access SARC and be examined, have her forensic samples stored anonymously and then have the option of involving the police at a later stage if she wishes.

Another option is to have anonymous testing of samples and anonymous sharing of information with the police.

Even if she declines to go to a SARC or have police involvement, you must ensure you still address all her other needs as detailed below.

STIs and PEP: you will be expected to demonstrate a knowledge of PEPSE and eligibility for this.

GUM follow-up: for STI testing and knowledge of window periods for different STIs is important. Don't forget to mention hepatitis B prophylaxis.

Emergency contraception: in this particular case, she is on the combined pill with good compliance and therefore does not need emergency contraception.

Support and counselling with appropriate signposting to relevant websites and services. Leaflets can be given.

SKILLS BEING ASSESSED:

This OSCE will be assessing your ability to show empathy and approach history taking in a sensitive manner. Communication and data gathering skills, as well as knowledge of PEPSE, the role of a SARC and window periods for STI testing are important components of this OSCE station.

SUGGESTED READING:

BASHH, *UK guideline for the use of HIV post-exposure prophylaxis following sexual exposure*, 2015.

BASHH, *UK national guidelines on the management of adult and adolescent complainants of sexual assault*, 2012.

OSCE Scenario Two

INFORMATION FOR THE DOCTOR:

Laura is 49 years old and has been struggling with hot flushes. She attends clinic wanting to know what to do. She would like to try HRT but has read things about it that say it is harmful. She has been married for 25 years and has 2 children.

BP – 120/80mmHg

BMI – 33

INFORMATION FOR PATIENT:

You are Laura and you are 49 years old. You have attended today because you have been having troublesome hot flushes for the past 6 months. You have heard that HRT can help with these symptoms, but you are worried because some of the information you have read about HRT has frightened you.

You would like advice.

Your ideas: you feel that the hot flushes are a sign that you are approaching the menopause. You are considering HRT, but recent information you have read online makes you wonder if commencing HRT is a good idea.

Your concerns: you have read that it is possible to have a blood clot in your legs or lungs with HRT and that it can give you breast cancer. Your mother had breast cancer, so this is a particular worry for you.

Your expectations: you would like advice about whether starting HRT at your age is safe.

Information to reveal if asked:

You have been considering HRT because you are having troublesome hot flushes, lasting 3–4 minutes each time and occurring with variable frequency throughout the day. The associated night sweats have been disturbing your sleep and making you feel tired during the day.

You are still having periods but you are aware that these symptoms may indicate that you are close to the menopause. You have been married for 25 years and have two children (normal deliveries). You are sexually active and use condoms for contraception. You have had no other partners and do not have any vaginal or urinary symptoms.

Your periods have changed in the past year. You now have a 25 day cycle, with the bleeding lasting for 10 days instead of your previous 5/28 day pattern. Your periods are much heavier and you often pass clots and you have had flooding.

You had a mammogram recently, which was normal. All cervical smear tests have been normal, you don't smoke and have a glass of wine occasionally. You do drink around 5 cups of coffee a day, but are trying to reduce this. You have no medical or surgical history of note and are fit and well. You are not on any medication and have no allergies.

Your mother had breast cancer and information you have read says that HRT increases the risk of breast cancer and also the risk of developing a blood clot in the leg or lung. This has made you very anxious and you are now questioning whether you should even be considering HRT.

TAKING A FOCUSED HISTORY:

Introduce yourself, confirm details.

Establish ICE – Ideas, Concerns and Expectations
- Why has she come to see you today?
- What is worrying her?
- What are her expectations from this consultation?

Explain that you will need to ask her some questions to see how best to help her.

History:
Presenting complaint
- **What** symptoms has she been getting?
  - Duration and severity of symptoms?
  - Sexually active? Regular partner?
  - Other partners? Contraception?
  - Vaginal dryness?
  - Any urinary symptoms?
  - Any unscheduled bleeding?
- **Menstrual history**: current pattern of bleeding?
  - If heavy, any clots, flooding?
  - Previous cycles?
  - Intermenstrual or post-coital bleeding?
- **Gynaecological history**
- **Contraception**
- **Medical history**: including breast cancer, liver disease, hypertension, VTE
- **Medication**: prescribed/over the counter/herbal remedies
- **Screening**: cytology, mammograms
- **Social history**: caffeine, alcohol, smoking, drug use
- **Family history**: breast cancer, VTE, osteoporosis
- **Examination**: BP and BMI already given

MANAGEMENT:

1. Heavy menstrual bleeding at this age would require investigation, i.e. ultrasound scan and an endometrial biopsy.
2. Lifestyle measures for helping menopausal symptoms – in this case reducing caffeine, benefits of a high calcium diet, exercise and weight loss.
3. Explain advantages of HRT at this age – beneficial effect on symptoms as well as on her bones and possibly cardiovascular system.

4. Address risks with HRT – VTE. Other risks are dependent upon an individual risk assessment following NICE CG23.

   Explain about the advantages of using a transdermal preparation in her case due to her BMI (VTE risk). No increase in risk over and above the risk that she has due to her weight. The lifelong risk of breast cancer is high for all women (1:8) and there is no increase in risk below the age of 60 (0.1% increase).
   Reassure her that a family history of breast cancer does not mean that HRT is contraindicated for her although she may be more likely to develop the disease. The end mortality is the same whether or not women take HRT.

5. Options for HRT:

   Mirena and oestrogen transdermally

   Consider a Mirena IUS (LNG 52mg) which would not only be of benefit to manage her heavy menstrual bleeding, but would also provide endometrial protection and contraception.

   As BMI>30, offer a transdermal oestrogen preparation, e.g. patch or gel; this is associated with least risk.

   Alternatively, if she does not want an IUS, she could have **sequential HRT** transdermally, but would need to continue with contraception.

   If Laura's symptoms were confined to the urogenital tract, she could use local oestrogen therapy. There are a variety of options including oestradiol pessaries (10mcg daily for 2 weeks then twice weekly for as long as needed), oestriol creams and Estring (a synthetic ring with a reservoir of oestrogen in its core, which is slowly released over a 3 month period).

6. Alternatives to HRT:

   Non-hormonal pharmacological treatments: clonidine, SSRIs, gabapentin.

   Non-pharmacological therapies: phytoestrogens, black cohosh, vitamin E, evening primrose oil.

   Lifestyle modifications: BMI – weight loss, smoking cessation, alcohol – reduction in intake, exercise.

7. Complementary therapies: acupuncture, yoga, Pilates, aromatherapy.

   Review: if investigations are normal and she agrees to commence HRT, explain that you will review her in 3 months and annually thereafter.

Mention that it is not unusual to get some irregular bleeding in the first 6 months, but if persistent this would require further investigation.

Information:
- Websites, e.g. www.menopausematters.co.uk
- Leaflet, e.g. *HRT Myths Uncovered*; available at bit.do/RG-1

SKILLS BEING ASSESSED:

This station tests your ability to communicate effectively and to address the concerns of the patient. You need to demonstrate thorough history taking skills and knowledge of menopause and its associated symptoms. You should be able to discuss the options for management including available preparations, benefits and risks of HRT, alternative and complementary therapies.

SUGGESTED READING:

NICE, *Menopause: diagnosis and management*. CG23, 2015.

OSCE Scenario Three

INFORMATION FOR THE DOCTOR:

Charlotte is 34 years old. She has come to see you today for contraception and mentions she has had infrequent, heavy periods for the past 2 years. She is bothered by excess hair growth on her face, which she has been removing by waxing.

INFORMATION FOR THE PATIENT:

You are Charlotte and you are 34 years old. You have attended clinic today requesting contraception because you are in a new relationship. You have noticed that your periods have become heavier and infrequent over the past couple of years, with bleeding occurring about three times a year.

Your ideas: you know that your periods should be more regular. When your period doesn't come, you worry that you could be pregnant and you would like contraception.

Your concerns: you worry that there is something wrong and that is why your periods have become infrequent. You are concerned that the lack of regular bleeding may be harmful for you.

Your expectations: you expect to receive contraception today and also advice about your heavy, infrequent periods and the best way to manage them.

Information to reveal if asked:

Your periods have become heavier over the past 2 years and you pass clots and have flooding too. You don't mind the fact that you bleed infrequently, but worry in case it may be having a harmful effect on your body. You have noticed hair growth on your face and neck over the past year and wonder if everything is related.

You started a new relationship with your partner Matt a month ago. You are currently using condoms effectively, but would like a more reliable method of contraception. Your last STI screen was 2 years ago and was normal.

You have joined a weight loss programme recently to try to reduce your weight. You have 2 children aged 12 and 8 years, both born by normal delivery and your family is complete. Your smear tests are up to date and have always been normal. You have no medical or surgical history of note. Your mother had a DVT aged 42 years. You don't smoke or drink alcohol and have never used recreational drugs.

If the candidate offers to check your BP and BMI, give them a card stating:

BP – 126/80mmHg

BMI – 39

TAKING A FOCUSED HISTORY:

Introduce yourself and confirm details, discuss confidentiality.

Establish ICE – Ideas, Concerns, Expectations
- Why has she come to see you today?
- What is worrying her?
- What are her expectations from this consultation?

History:
Presenting problem: request for contraception/infrequent heavy periods.
- Duration of bleeding problems?
- How heavy is the bleeding? Clots? Flooding?
- How frequently does her period come?
- Any other symptoms she has noticed?
- Any weight gain/loss?
- Any excess facial or body hair growth?
- Has she thought about which method of contraception she would like?
- Stress?

Menstrual history: LMP, previous cycles, intermenstrual bleeding, post-coital bleeding?

Obstetric history: parity, modes of delivery?

Gynaecological history: previous diagnoses, cytology up to date and normal?

Sexual history: partner? Regular/casual?
- Duration of relationship?
- Any other partners? Condoms?
- Last STI screen

Contraception

Medical history: check if fit and well

Medication: prescribed/over the counter/herbal remedies

Family history: VTE, other significant history

Social history: smoking, alcohol, recreational drug use

EXAMINATION: BP, BMI, STI screen

MANAGEMENT:

Based on the clinical picture, the diagnosis here would be PCOS.

1. Offer a transvaginal ultrasound scan to assess ovaries and endometrium.
2. Lifestyle changes – weight loss, diet modification and exercise. You should be able to discuss the important role of weight loss in the management of PCOS.
3. Because Charlotte is seeking reliable long-term contraception, an IUS could be offered to her (provides contraception and endometrial protection). Her raised BMI and family history of VTE mean that combined hormonal contraception choices (pills, patches and vaginal rings) are contraindicated.
4. For the facial hair, cosmetic options can be sought, e.g. laser treatment, Vaniqa cream.

SKILLS BEING ASSESSED:

This station is testing your ability to carry out effective data gathering and assesses your knowledge of the clinical presentation and management of PCOS.

SUGGESTED READING:

Duncan, A guide to understanding polycystic ovary syndrome (PCOS). *J Fam Plann Reprod Health Care*, 2014;40:217.

RCOG, *Long-term consequences of polycystic ovary syndrome*. GTG33, 2014.

UKMEC 2016.

OSCE Scenario Four

INFORMATION FOR THE DOCTOR:

Rachel is 26 years old and attends for contraception. She mentions that she had unprotected sex with a casual partner 80 hours ago.

BP – 120/76mmHg

BMI – 25

INFORMATION FOR THE PATIENT:

You are Rachel and you are 26 years old and you are requesting contraception. You had unprotected sex with a casual partner 80 hours ago.

Your ideas: you know that you need effective contraception because you have had a pregnancy recently and don't want to get pregnant again in the near future.

Your concerns: you are worried that you might be pregnant from the sex you had 80 hours ago.

Your expectations: you expect to receive a contraceptive method to start today.

Information to reveal if asked:

You had an ectopic pregnancy (in your fallopian tube), which was treated medically (methotrexate), 14 days ago. Blood tests have shown this treatment was successful. That was your first pregnancy and you found the whole process, from diagnosis to treatment, emotionally draining.

You don't think you could face getting pregnant again and are feeling angry at yourself for having consensual sex without a condom 80 hours ago and putting yourself at risk of a pregnancy. The person you had sex with is a white, local male and you met him through mutual friends.

Until recently you were in a relationship with a regular male partner for 2 years but you broke up a month ago. You have had one smear test in the past, which was normal. Your last STI screen was 2 weeks ago and was normal. You have not had a proper period yet following the ectopic pregnancy. Your previous cycles were regular and 28 days apart, with bleeding lasting 5 days.

You do not have any medical, surgical or family history of note. You are not on any medication and don't have any allergies.

You smoke 10 cigarettes a day, but don't drink alcohol or use recreational drugs.

Ideally you would prefer a long acting reversible method of contraception today.

TAKING A FOCUSED HISTORY:

Introduce yourself, confirm details and explain confidentiality.

Establish ICE – Ideas, Concerns and Expectations
- Why has she come to see you today?
- What is worrying her?
- What are her expectations from this consultation?

History:
Presenting complaint: details of recent ectopic pregnancy
- Confirm treatment for the ectopic pregnancy
- UPSI:
    o When?
    o Any other episodes?
    o Consensual
    o Casual partner: male/female, ethnicity

Sexual history: number of other partners in last 12 months
- Condom usage?
- Previous STIs

Obstetric history: other pregnancies and outcomes including modes of delivery

Menstrual history: previous cycles, bleeding pattern

Gynaecology history: including cytology

Medical history: including VTE, liver disease, migraines, hypertension

Medication: prescribed/over the counter/herbal remedies

Social history: smoking, alcohol, recreational drugs

Allergies?

EXAMINATION: BP, BMI (already given)

MANAGEMENT:

It is important that you are familiar with the most recently published FSRH Emergency contraception guidance and the Post-pregnancy contraception guideline. The latter highlights the importance of contraception following ectopic pregnancy.

Tip 1

Emergency contraception OSCE stations can be particularly tricky. UPSI may be a 'hidden agenda' which may only be revealed during the course of the history taking.

Tip 2

There may be props in the station such as calendars and leaflets, which you should look out for and use.

As Rachel has been treated with methotrexate for her ectopic pregnancy, she should be advised to use **effective contraception during and for at least 3 months after treatment** in view of the teratogenic effects of methotrexate.

Emergency contraception is indicated if unprotected sexual intercourse takes place more than 5 days after methotrexate administration or surgical treatment of ectopic pregnancy.

In this OSCE scenario, the patient had UPSI 14 days after taking methotrexate. She presented for help 80 hours afterwards and is therefore eligible for any of the emergency contraceptive options. Due to the risk of teratogenesis, she should be advised to have the most effective option, a copper IUD. This can be left *in situ* to provide reliable ongoing contraception if she agrees.

Counselling for Cu-IUD: benefits, risks, insertion procedure and self-checking of threads should be explained to her.

Antibiotic cover for STI should be considered and screening offered with repeat testing 2 weeks after the UPSI (window period) for chlamydia and gonorrhoea and at 8 weeks for blood-borne viruses.

If she declines an IUD, you should discuss the emergency hormonal options, in order of efficacy: UPA-EC followed by LNG-EC:

- UPA-EC is the next most effective method, but commencing hormonal contraception needs to be delayed for 5 days during which time there is an ongoing risk of pregnancy and condoms must be used until reliable contraception becomes effective.
- Because it is less effective, LNG-EC would not be recommended due to the risk of teratogenesis if conception did occur. LNG-EC is licensed for use up to 72 hours after UPSI. If taken more than 96 hours after UPSI, evidence suggests LNG-EC is not effective. Hormonal contraception can be quick-started immediately after LNG-EC, with additional precautions until it becomes effective.

A pregnancy test should be carried out in 3–4 weeks following EHC.

Advice on safe sex and smoking cessation.

Offer condoms.

Information: leaflets, website (www.fpa.org.uk/contraception-help/emergency-contraception)

SKILLS BEING ASSESSED:

This OSCE station looks at your data gathering skills, communication skills, ability to formulate a management plan, and also assesses your knowledge of management of ectopic pregnancy and emergency contraception.

SUGGESTED READING:

RCOG, *Diagnosis and management of ectopic pregnancy.* GTG21, 2016.

NICE, *Ectopic pregnancy and miscarrriage: diagnosis and initial management in early pregnancy of ectopic pregnancy and miscarriage.* CG154, 2012.

FSRH, *CEU clinical guidance: Emergency contraception.* March 2017.

FSRH, *CEU clinical guidance: Contraception after pregnancy.* January 2017.

OSCE Scenario Five

INFORMATION FOR THE DOCTOR:

Julie, a 56-year-old postmenopausal woman attends clinic complaining of vaginal dryness. She seems anxious and embarrassed.

BP – 110/76mmHg

BMI – 29

INFORMATION FOR THE PATIENT:

You are 56 years old and have attended clinic today feeling anxious and embarrassed. You have been struggling with symptoms of vaginal dryness for the past 2 years.

Your ideas: you feel the vaginal dryness is related to the menopause.

Your concerns: the dryness has been causing you pain and discomfort during sex and you worry that this will impact on your relationship with your partner.

Your expectations: you expect to get some treatment today to help with your symptoms.

Information to reveal if asked:

The vaginal dryness has got worse since you stopped having periods 2 years ago. You have had no treatment to date. You have been married for 26 years and have 2 grown-up children, both of whom were born by normal delivery. You have not had sex with your husband for more than 12 months due to the pain and discomfort you feel on penetration.

Your most troublesome symptom, but the one you have been too embarrassed to mention, is that of needing to go the toilet to pass urine frequently. You noticed this after your menopause and the symptoms have got worse over the past year. On occasion, you have struggled to reach the toilet in time and have had 'accidents' (episodes of leakage) so you now wear pads. You don't leak on coughing or sneezing and do not have any burning or pain when passing urine. You need to get up at least twice a night to go to the toilet and this disturbs your sleep. You do not have any bowel problems and have never had any faecal incontinence. You are fit and well, with no significant medical or surgical history. You don't smoke or drink alcohol other than at social occasions. You have no gynaecological history of note. You do enjoy drinking tea – you have around 6 cups a day. You have no allergies and are not on any medication. You have had no bleeding since your last menstrual period.

TAKING A FOCUSED HISTORY:

Introduce yourself and confirm details.

Establish ICE – Ideas, Concerns, Expectations
- Why has she come to see you today?
- What is worrying her?*
- What are her expectations from this consultation?

  Tip:
  Acknowledge non-verbal cues.

History:
Presenting issue:
- Duration of symptoms
- How troublesome are her symptoms?
- Has she tried anything for the dryness yet?
- Is she sexually active?
- Length of relationship?
  - o Any impact on relationship?
  - o Impact on day to day life?
- Any urinary or bowel problems?
  - o Leakage on coughing or sneezing?
  - o Does she use pads? How many a day?
  - o Nocturia?
  - o Burning or pain on passing urine?
  - o Any accidents, i.e. leakage before reaching the toilet? Faecal incontinence?

Obstetric history: parity, modes of delivery

Gynaecology history: including cytology

Menstrual history: age of menopause, postmenopausal or postcoital bleeding?

Medical history: including any cardiac, neurological problems, hypertension

Medication: antihypertensives? HRT? Over the counter/herbal remedies/prescribed medication?

Allergies?

Surgical history:

Family history:

Social history: smoking, alcohol, drugs, caffeine and tea intake

EXAMINATION: BMI, BP (results already given)
- General exam, including noting of any impairment of mobility
- Abdominal exam, including any abdominal masses or incisions from previous surgical intervention
- Vaginal exam, looking for signs of atrophy, ulceration, or prolapse

INVESTIGATIONS:
- Urine dipstick
- Quality of life questionnaire
- Voiding diary for 3 days (documenting fluid intake, output and leakage)
- Portable bladder scan to check post void residual volume measurement

MANAGEMENT:

It is important that you are aware of the management of all types of urinary incontinence. The symptom profile should guide you towards a particular diagnosis, e.g. urge incontinence (UI).

In this case the initial management would include:
1. Lifestyle changes, e.g. reducing intake of tea/coffee, weight loss
2. Bladder retraining
3. Antimuscarinic drugs
4. Oestradiol vaginal pessaries (Vagifem 10mcg × 2/week)
5. Vaginal moisturisers, e.g. Hyalofemme

Information: leaflets, website (www.menopausematters.co.uk)

SKILLS BEING ASSESSED:

This is a typical OSCE scenario where there is a hidden agenda. Your communication skills as well as your data gathering capabilities and ability to formulate an appropriate management plan are being assessed. The patient has attended regarding vaginal dryness, but may divulge issues such as psychosexual problems as a result of dyspareunia, secondary to vaginal dryness or as in this case, urinary incontinence.

You should be able to ask questions and discuss these issues sensitively.

SUGGESTED READING:

NICE, *Urinary incontinence in women: management. CG171*, 2016.

OSCE Scenario Six

INFORMATION FOR THE DOCTOR:

You are the lead doctor in a busy community clinic. You are new to the service, but have heard that this particular clinic frequently runs behind schedule because 'the nurses are very slow'. There are two nurses today offering appointments in addition to your appointments. A receptionist is booking patients in on arrival. There is a patient in the waiting room who is being disruptive. She is angry due to the waiting time. Although this patient is not on your list, you decide that it would be best for you to see her now to avoid further disruption.

INFORMATION FOR THE PATIENT:

You are Mrs Whittaker and are 35 years old. You attended clinic for a smear test today but have been waiting for an hour. This has made you very frustrated and angry and you made that quite clear to the receptionist by raising your voice and threatening to walk out. You had heard that this particular clinic is very busy, but you didn't realise how long you would have to wait.

Your ideas: you think it's ridiculous that patients have to wait so long to be seen. What is the point of having an appointment time if staff won't keep to it?

Your concerns: you worry that you will 'lose your nerve' and not have the smear today. You have taken the whole day off work today for this and can't keep taking time off.

Your expectations: you expect to have the smear test today and would like an explanation as to why you have had to wait so long to be seen when you have an appointment with one of the nurses.

Information to reveal if asked:

You are 35 years old and have never had a cervical smear test. You were in an abusive relationship for 12 years in which you often felt pressurised into having sex. This has led to psychosexual issues and you are seeking help through psychosexual counselling. You had to mentally build yourself up to attend for your first smear test today and that is why the long waiting time has been incredibly frustrating for you. You worry that you will lose your nerve and leave the clinic today without having the smear done. You feel angry at all the staff for the delay.

You are currently not in a relationship. You left your abusive partner 3 years ago. You had to involve the police because he was mentally and physically abusive and you now have no contact with him. You have never had any children and have no medical, surgical or family history of note. You are not on any medication and have no allergies. You don't smoke and have alcohol only occasionally. You had an STI screen at the end of your relationship, which was negative.

TAKING A FOCUSED HISTORY:

Introduce yourself, confirm details and explain confidentiality.

Establish ICE – Ideas, Concerns, Expectations
- Why has she come to see you today?
- What is worrying her?
- What are her expectations from this consultation?

Tip 1
This OSCE may be given as a written station initially, followed by a viva with the examiner.

Tip 2
There are different aspects to this station - identify the various issues relating to each aspect.

History:
Presenting issue: Is she up to date with her smear tests? If not, why not?
- Has she ever had a smear test?
- Result of any previous smear tests?

Obstetric history: parity, miscarriages, abortions, ectopic pregnancies?

Gynaecology history: contraception? LMP, cycle, any unscheduled bleeding?

Sexual history: partner? Regular/casual? Duration of relationship?
- Any other partners?
  - Condoms?
  - STI screen?

Medical history: check if fit and well

Medication: prescribed/over the counter/herbal remedies?

Social history: smoking, alcohol, recreational drug use?

EXAMINATION: offer BP, BMI, smear test today

MANAGEMENT:

Patient aspect
You or your assistant should:
- Apologise to other patients in the waiting room and explain that the clinic is running late.

- Give them the option of rebooking their appointment, if they are unable to wait.

Disruptive patient

Introduce yourself:

- Apologise for the clinic running late and the waiting time.
- Offer to speak to her separately in another room (but preferably with a chaperone).
- If the patient is abusive and disruptive, you may need to call security or the police.
- Explain that you will look into the delay and see where changes can be made.
- Check if she still wants her smear test done today and encourage her to do so.

Explain the nature of the test, possible results and how she will receive them. Be reassuring.

Clinician aspect

Efficiency of the clinic

- Look at the number of patients on lists for the nurses and doctors. Do the appointment times correspond with the FSRH service specification standards?
- Which clinic(s) is running behind?
- Whose list is this patient on and what was the delay?
- Are the patients on the nurses' lists appropriately booked for their skill set?
- Look at your own clinic and ascertain if and why it is running late – is it a complex contraception clinic necessitating longer appointment times, e.g. removal of deep implants?
- Ratio of new patients to review patients.
- Time allocated for each consultation.
- A full debrief with all clinic staff including the receptionist should take place at the end of clinic.

The discussion should focus on why the clinic recurrently runs behind schedule and the possible reasons for this and potential solutions.

Review of data provided by the receptionist will inform the most effective way of resolving the current problem. This should reduce stress experienced by both patients and clinicians.

Any trend of delay noticed with a particular staff member?

- If so, arrange to speak to that particular staff member separately. You may identify training issues or health/personal issues.
- Can offer support, further training, supervised sessions or referral to occupational health.

Other issues

- An incident report/Datix form should be filled out in relation to this event.
- The patient may want to make a complaint - provide details for PALS.

- Inform service manager, nursing line manager (if different) and clinical lead.
- It is sensible to write a statement yourself for your own records because it can be difficult to remember details if there is a delay in a potential complaint being processed.

Review clinic template to reduce delays:
- Reduce the number of appointments?
- Consider increasing appointment times for complex procedures.
- Look at booking processes.

OSCE Scenario Seven

INFORMATION FOR THE DOCTOR:

Aisha is 27 years old and attends your clinic feeling quite angry. She had an implant fitted 6 weeks ago following an abortion. She thinks it was inserted in her left arm. She is unable to feel the implant and wants to know if there is a problem.

INFORMATION FOR THE PATIENT:

You are Aisha and you are 27 years old. You attend the clinic feeling very angry because you are unable to feel the contraceptive implant which was fitted in your left arm following an abortion 6 weeks ago.

Your ideas: you know that you should be able to feel the implant. Because you cannot feel it, you think it was put in incorrectly by someone 'who didn't know what they were doing'. You don't want to have another unplanned pregnancy and feel very worried because you have been relying on this as contraception.

Your concerns: you are worried that the implant has 'gone missing'.

Your expectations: you expect to find out what has happened and where the implant is.

Information to reveal if asked:

You had your implant fitted by a nurse in the local sexual health service 6 weeks ago. It was fitted in your left arm, 3 days after a medical abortion. You and the nurse were unable to feel the implant after fitting but she assumed that was because of the local anaesthetic that she had injected.

You have not 'played' with the implant following fitting and don't remember any problems occurring during the fitting. Your arm was externally rotated and flexed during the fitting and you have not had any bleeding for the past month. Unfortunately you have lost your implant card.

You have been in a relationship with your male partner for the last 3 years. During this time you have had no other partners. You have a 2 year old child, born by normal delivery. You had a medical abortion 6 weeks ago because you did not feel ready to have another baby. A full STI screen was done at the time of abortion and you were told the results were negative. You last had sex 3 weeks ago.

You have had one smear test in the past, which was normal, and have no significant medical or surgical history of note. You don't smoke or drink alcohol and have never used recreational drugs.

You are not on any medications and have no allergies.

If the doctor offers to check your BP and BMI, hand them a card saying

BP – 110/70mmHg

BMI – 19

TAKING A FOCUSED HISTORY:

Introduce yourself and confirm patient details, explain confidentiality

Establish ICE – Ideas, Concerns, Expectations
- Why has she come to see you today?
- What is worrying her?
- What are her expectations from this consultation?

History:
Presenting complaint – when and where was the implant fitted?
- Does she still have her implant card? (this often has helpful details)
- In which arm was the implant fitted?
- Does she recall feeling for the implant after fitting?
- Did the fitter confirm that it was palpable post-insertion?
- Has she ever been able to feel it?
- Had she 'played' with the implant at all?
- Does she recall the position of her arm during fitting?
- Current bleeding pattern?

Obstetric history: parity, recent abortion

Gynaecology history: cytology up to date and normal?

Sexual history: partner? Regular/casual?
- Duration of relationship?
- Any other partners? Condoms?
- Check if STI screen done at time of abortion and if results received.

Medical history: check if fit and well

Medication: prescribed/over the counter/herbal remedies?

Social history: smoking, alcohol, recreational drug use

EXAMINATION:
- Need to examine both arms fully
- BP, BMI
- Pregnancy test

MANAGEMENT:

In this situation, the actor may initially be angry and it is important to communicate effectively with them to calm them down so that you can complete all aspects of the station.

Acknowledge that her frustration is understandable.

Review clinic notes from the implant fitting procedure (if possible). Explain the rationale for doing a pregnancy test today (risk of pregnancy in association with non-insertion).

Explain that an ultrasound scan is required to locate the implant. (If not seen on the ultrasound scan, then an X-ray of both arms and the chest should be performed.) If neither of these imaging techniques shows that the implant is present, a blood test to measure the hormone released by the implant (etonogestrel) will need to be done.

You should be aware of the possibility of intravascular insertions (see CEU update 2016), hence the need to do a chest X-ray.

You can offer to discuss and then feed back to the person who fitted her implant.

The other issue to mention is ongoing contraception. Until the implant is located, it is important to use additional contraception. She may choose to quick start a method today, based on a risk assessment.

SKILLS ASSESSED:

This station is looking at your communication skills, in particular your ability to deal with a difficult patient. Your knowledge base and ability to formulate an appropriate management plan are also covered.

SUGGESTED READING:

FSRH, *CEU guidance: Progestogen-only implants.* 2014.

FSRH, *CEU statement: Intravascular insertion of Nexplanon.* 2016.

OSCE Scenario Eight

INFORMATION FOR THE DOCTOR:

Hannah is 15 years old and has come to see you in clinic on her own. She has been taking the combined pill for contraception, but thinks she may have missed a few pills. She did a pregnancy test at home which was positive and she is adamant that she cannot continue with the pregnancy.

BP today – 116/70mmHg

BMI – 23

INFORMATION FOR THE PATIENT:

You are Hannah; you are 15 years old and have come to clinic today feeling very worried. You have been taking the combined pill for contraception and think you might have missed a few. You did a pregnancy test and it was positive. You don't feel ready to have a baby and want some advice.

Your ideas: you have found out that you are pregnant and know that you are not ready to have a baby.

Your concerns: you think your partner will be angry and break up with you if he finds out that you are pregnant.

Your expectations: you expect to be told about what treatment options there are for an unwanted pregnancy.

Information to reveal if asked:

You have been with your partner, Steve, for 6 months. He was the first person you ever had sex with and he convinced you to take the combined pill for contraception. He is 20 years old and you feel he treats you nicely as he buys you a lot of things like the new trainers you are wearing today. He hasn't ever forced you to have sex but you don't like saying no to him as you feel you should keep him happy.

Steve can get angry sometimes and has hit you a few times over the past few months. You feel that you deserved it though as you made 'silly mistakes' which would 'wind him up'. You don't see your friends any more because he doesn't like them. You live with your mum but she is unaware of the relationship. You are scared of Steve's reaction if he found out you had become pregnant because he told you to take the pill and you forgot some. You feel it's all your fault and are keen to use effective contraception 'once this is all over'.

You have no medical, surgical or family history of note.

You are not on any medication and have no allergies.

You smoke 10 cigarettes a day and have alcohol with Steve at weekends, but not too much as you don't really like the taste. You have never used drugs.

You have never had an STI screen before but agree to having one done.

TAKING A FOCUSED HISTORY:

Introduce yourself, confirm details and explain confidentiality policy and any limits.

Establish ICE – Ideas, Concerns, Expectations
- Why has she come to see you today?
- What is worrying her?
- What are her expectations from this consultation?

  Tip 1
  Be aware that you may be given non-verbal cues by the actor and you should acknowledge these in your consultation.

  Tip 2
  Whilst asking the above questions, you are also determining Fraser competency.

Explain that you will need to ask her some questions to see how best to help her.

History:
- Does she have a current partner? How old is he?
- Aware of pregnancy? If not, any reason?
- Duration of relationship?
- Other partners in the last 12 months?
- Condom use? Method of contraception?
- Consensual sex? Coercion? Any gifts in exchange for sex?
- Domestic abuse – mental or physical? Does she feel safe?
- Support: who knows about the pregnancy? Does she have any support at home?
- Does she have a social/key worker (identifies vulnerable child/adult)?

Menstrual history: LMP/withdrawal bleed, normal cycles, problematic bleeding?
- When did she first have a positive pregnancy test?

Obstetric history: parity, miscarriages, abortions
- Reason for abortion?

Medical history: including migraine, VTE

Social history: smoking, alcohol, drug use

Future contraception:
- Any method she is keen to try?
- Is she aware of LARC?

EXAMINATION: BP, BMI (results already given)

INVESTIGATIONS:

- STI screening
- Transvaginal scan to determine gestation

MANAGEMENT :

- Application of Fraser guidelines for competence.
- Explain that there are various methods of abortion depending on the gestation.
  - o Medical method using mifepristone and then misoprostol
  - o Surgical method until 14 weeks of gestation – MVA under local anaesthetic
  - o Surgical method until 14 weeks of gestation – under general anaesthetic
- Show awareness of what each method entails, risks and failure rates of each method.
- Explain that it is illegal to have sex at 15 (below the age of consent).
  - o There are safeguarding issues – older partner, abusive relationship, coercion and exploitation.
  - o Explain that you will need to report this to the relevant agencies for her safety.
  - o You should be aware of the different agencies involved including police, children's safeguarding.
- Safe sex and STI prevention – explain about condom usage in addition to reliable contraception. Offer LARC.

Information: websites, leaflets (contraception (FPA leaflets), abortion), Helpline numbers.

SKILLS BEING ASSESSED:

This station tests not only your communication skills but also your ability to demonstrate effective data gathering to reveal the hidden agenda. Key points being looked at will be a sensitive approach to your history taking and an empathetic manner. You should be able to formulate a management plan for the issues identified in this station and show a thorough understanding of the topics.

SUGGESTED READING:

RCOG, *The care of women requesting induced abortion*. EBCG 7, 2011.

OSCE Scenario Nine

INFORMATION FOR THE DOCTOR:

Gemma is 36 years old and has come to see you to discuss contraception. She had a baby 19 days ago and is currently bottle-feeding. She smokes 20 cigarettes a day and is in a relationship.

INFORMATION FOR PATIENT:

You are Gemma and you are 36 years old. You have attended today to discuss contraception. You had your first baby 19 days ago by emergency caesarean section and had a postpartum haemorrhage at that time. You are currently bottle-feeding your baby.

You smoke 20 cigarettes a day and are in a relationship. You are very quiet and make little eye contact.

You were hoping to get the combined patch to start today because you have used that in the past and liked the regular bleeding pattern.

Your ideas: you are feeling very tired because you had a baby 19 days ago and are going through what all new mothers do.

Your concerns: you don't think you are doing a very good job as a mother and wonder how you will care for the baby.

Your expectations: you would like to get the combined patch today for contraception because you have found having a baby very difficult and do not want to get pregnant again.

Information to reveal if asked:

You have had a regular partner for the last 2 years and he is the father of the baby. He has a busy job so is away a lot of the time. Your parents live in Scotland so you don't see them much.

You had an emergency caesarean section for foetal distress and the baby had to spend 2 days in the neonatal ICU. You had to stay in hospital for longer than other mums and struggled to breastfeed. This made you feel low and inadequate.

Since the baby has been born, you feel tearful, struggle with sleeping and have lost your appetite. You have struggled to bond with the baby and feel exhausted although you have had no thoughts of harming the baby or yourself. You seem to be tired all the time and have lost interest in doing things you used to enjoy.

You hadn't seen your GP about this because you thought this is what all new mums go through, but you now accept that you will need to see them for some help and support.

Your previous menstrual cycles have been regular and all past cytology has been normal. You have no medical history of note, no allergies and are not on any medication. There is no significant family history.

If an examination to check your BP and BMI is mentioned by the candidate, you may give them a card with the following readings:

BP – 118/70mmHg

BMI – 37

TAKING A FOCUSED HISTORY:

Introduce yourself and confirm details, explain confidentiality

Establish ICE – Ideas, Concerns, Expectations
- Why has she come to see you today?
- What is worrying her?
- What are her expectations from this consultation?

Tip 1
Be aware that you may be given non-verbal cues by the actor. Here you are told the patient seems quiet and makes little eye contact. You should acknowledge this because it will help reveal any hidden agenda and you can formulate your questions accordingly.

History:
Presenting issue:
- Acknowledge non-verbal cues and respond accordingly.
- Any particular contraceptive method she was hoping for? Reason?
- Preferred bleeding pattern?
- Relationship: partner? Is he father of this baby?
   o Regular/casual? Length of relationship?
   o Supportive? Any issues of domestic abuse?
   o STI risk?
- Mental health: how is she coping?
   o Does she have support at home? Family & friends?

Tip 2 – quick verbal screen for depression
In the past month has she felt down, depressed, hopeless?
Does she feel she has lost interest in things she used to enjoy?
Sleep, appetite
Feelings towards the baby – bonding, harm
Thoughts of self-harm, hearing voices, hallucinations

Obstetric history: parity and modes of delivery, miscarriages, abortions
- How was her recent pregnancy and delivery?
- Any problems, e.g. PPH, pre-eclampsia?
- Other children? How many? Do they live with her?

Menstrual history: previous cycles, post-coital or intermenstrual bleeding?

Gynaecology history: cytology – up to date? Past cytology normal?

Medical history: hypertension, migraines, VTE, liver or cardiac problems?

Medication: over the counter/herbal remedies/prescribed medication?

Family history: VTE and other relevant history

Social history: smoking, alcohol, recreational drugs, FGM

EXAMINATION: BP, BMI (results already given)

MANAGEMENT:

Gemma is a postnatal woman who seems quiet and is showing little eye contact. You should be aware of postnatal depression and how to ask questions sensitively to explore this. Acknowledging the non-verbal cues early in the consultation will reveal this agenda.

You should be able to offer help/support depending upon the information you receive. Explain the importance of involving her GP in her care, accessing counselling services, midwife/health visitor.

- As she is not breastfeeding and is less than 3 weeks postnatal, with multiple risk factors for VTE (caesarean section, raised BMI, smoker), you should be aware that an IUD/IUS would be UKMEC3, whilst CHC would be UKMEC4.
- It is important to negotiate a shared management plan with Gemma and offer appropriate LARC or bridge with a POP if timing not appropriate, STI screening, condoms.
- Arrange a follow-up appointment.

Information: leaflets, websites (www.fpa.org.uk/sites/default/files/contraception-after-having-baby-your-guide.pdf, www.LAC-info.com)

SKILLS BEING ASSESSED:

This station tests not only your communication skills, but also your ability to use the data provided in the question to make a decision.

You need to demonstrate how to take a thorough history and how to broach a subject like postnatal depression in a sensitive manner.

Good communication
- Empathises with patient's concerns.
- Is systematic during history taking.
- Allows the patient time to express their thoughts fully.
- Discusses pros and cons of different contraceptive options and the risks of giving CHC methods today.
- Is able to discuss management plan for support and the rationale for involving GP, health visitor, etc. in a sensitive manner.

Poor communication

- Does not take a systematic history.
- Does not pick up verbal and non-verbal cues.
- Does not show empathy; shows hastiness in history taking and management without taking into account the patient's concerns and wishes.

SUGGESTED READING:

FSRH, *Guideline – Contraception after pregnancy*. January 2017.

NICE, *Antenatal and postnatal mental health*. CG192, 2014.

UKMEC 2016.

OSCE Scenario Ten

Andy is a 22-year-old student. He has recently come back from a holiday in Thailand and attends the clinic requesting an HIV test.

INFORMATION FOR THE PATIENT:

You are Andy, a 22-year-old student. You have recently returned to the UK following a 3 week trip to Thailand. During this time you had sex with a local male. You attend clinic today for an HIV test and look worried.

Your ideas: you are aware that not using a condom can put you at risk of infections.

Your concerns: you are worried that you may have been exposed to HIV and other infections and that you may have passed these on to your partner.

Your expectations: you expect to have an HIV test today.

Information to reveal if asked:

You have only ever had male partners and are currently in a relationship. You have been with your regular partner for a year and you normally use condoms with him.

You travelled alone to Thailand for a 3 week trip and only returned a week ago.

During your holiday you had anal sex (received) with a local man 2 weeks ago and did not use a condom. You are usually very careful and are now worried that you may have become infected with HIV and might have passed it on to your partner.

You have not been vaccinated against hepatitis B. The last time you had an STI screen was 6 months ago.

You do not have any symptoms like burning, pain in your testicles or any pain on passing urine.

You have never injected drugs and have never paid for sex.

You smoke 10 cigarettes a day and have occasional alcohol on the weekends.

You have no medical or surgical history of note and are not on any medication. You do not have any allergies.

TAKING A FOCUSED HISTORY:

Introduce yourself and confirm details, explain confidentiality.

Establish ICE – Ideas, Concerns, Expectations
- Why has he come to see you today?
- What is worrying him?
- What are his expectations from this consultation?

History:
Presenting issue: reason for requesting HIV test?
- Does he feel he has been at risk?
- Any symptoms: discharge, pain on passing urine, pain in his testicles, any lumps?
- When did he return from Thailand and what was the duration of the holiday?
- Any sex whilst on holiday in Thailand?
  - o If so, male or female partner?
  - o Type of sex (oral/anal): if anal sex, receptive or insertive?
  - o Ethnicity of partner?
  - o Condom used?
  - o Other sexual partners?

Sexual history: is he in a relationship? Casual/ regular partner? Male or female? Ethnicity?
- Type of sex and details regarding receptive or insertive anal sex, oral sex or both.
  - o Condom usage?
- Last STI screen including HIV test?
  - o Ever had an STI?
- Paid for sex?
- Drug use, including intravenous drug use?
- Has he ever been vaccinated against hepatitis B?

Medical history:
- Kidney, liver or bone disease?
- Hypertension? Diabetes? Raised cholesterol?

Medication: prescribed/over the counter/herbal remedies?

Social history: smoking, alcohol, drugs?

Allergies?

EXAMINATION:

- Urine test: chlamydia, gonorrhoea.
- HIV screen (POCT and a venous sample).
- Serum creatinine.
- Hepatitis B vaccination.
- Follow-up test if in window period.

MANAGEMENT:

- Andy has been having high risk sex, which increases his chances of acquiring an STI like HIV.
  - Has Andy considered the possibility that the test could be positive? Does he have support?
- If the test is positive, explain partner notification issues.
- The high risk sex was 2 weeks ago and therefore he is within the correct timeframe for urine testing for chlamydia and gonorrhoea.
  - How would he like to be informed of his results from the tests taken today?
  - Explain the window periods for STIs.
- You should be aware of both PEPSE and PrEP and when to offer.
  - PrEP is currently not available on the NHS. However, Andy could purchase it online or privately.
  - You should be aware of the 2 studies (PROUD, IPERGAY) which showed a large reduction in incidence of HIV when PrEP was given to men who have sex with men having anal sex without a condom.
  - **PrEP has 2 regimes: event-based or a daily regime.**
  - If Andy is interested in starting PrEP, then the above tests can be done and a follow-up appointment made in 1 month or 3 months after starting PrEP to ensure correct usage, assess any side-effects, and further testing as he is in the window period.
- Advise regarding future safe sex.

Information: leaflets and websites (www.iwantprepnow.co.uk).

SUGGESTED READING:

BASHH, *UK guideline for the use of HIV post-exposure prophylaxis following sexual exposure.* 2015.

BASHH, BHIVA, BIS, *UK national guidelines for HIV testing.* 2008.

BHIVA-BASHH, *Position statement on PrEP in the UK.* 2016.